STUDY GUIDE TO ACCOMPANY

Breastfeeding *and* Human Lactation

FOURTH EDITION

Mary-Margaret Coates, MS
Galactaguide
Wheat Ridge, Colorado

Jan Riordan, EdD, RN, IBCLC, FAAN
Professor
School of Nursing
Wichita State University
Wichita, Kansas

JONES AND BARTLETT PUBLISHERS
Sudbury, Massachusetts
BOSTON   TORONTO   LONDON   SINGAPORE

World Headquarters
Jones and Bartlett Publishers
40 Tall Pine Drive
Sudbury, MA 01776
978-443-5000
info@jbpub.com
www.jbpub.com

Jones and Bartlett Publishers
Canada
6339 Ormindale Way
Mississauga, Ontario L5V 1J2
Canada

Jones and Bartlett Publishers
International
Barb House, Barb Mews
London W6 7PA
United Kingdom

Jones and Bartlett's books and products are available through most bookstores and online booksellers. To contact Jones and Bartlett Publishers directly, call 800-832-0034, fax 978-443-8000, or visit our website, www.jbpub.com.

Substantial discounts on bulk quantities of Jones and Bartlett's publications are available to corporations, professional associations, and other qualified organizations. For details and specific discount information, contact the special sales department at Jones and Bartlett via the above contact information or send an email to specialsales@jbpub.com.

The authors, editor, and publisher have made every effort to provide accurate information. However, they are not responsible for errors, omissions, or for any outcomes related to the use of the contents of this book and take no responsibility for the use of the products and procedures described. Treatments and side effects described in this book may not be applicable to all people; likewise, some people may require a dose or experience a side effect that is not described herein. Drugs and medical devices are discussed that may have limited availability controlled by the Food and Drug Administration (FDA) for use only in a research study or clinical trial. Research, clinical practice, and government regulations often change the accepted standard in this field. When consideration is being given to use of any drug in the clinical setting, the health care provider or reader is responsible for determining FDA status of the drug, reading the package insert, and reviewing prescribing information for the most up-to-date recommendations on dose, precautions, and contraindications, and determining the appropriate usage for the product. This is especially important in the case of drugs that are new or seldom used.

Production Credits
Publisher: Kevin Sullivan
Acquisitions Editor: Emily Ekle
Acquisitions Editor: Amy Sibley
Associate Editor: Patricia Donnelly
Editorial Assistant: Rachel Shuster
Senior Production Editor: Carolyn F. Rogers
Marketing Manager: Rebecca Wasley
V.P., Manufacturing and Inventory Control: Therese Connell
Composition and Text Design: Auburn Associates, Inc.
Cover Design: Kristin E. Parker
Cover Image: Courtesy of Mary-Margaret Coates
Section 1 Opener Image: Courtesy of Jan Riordan
Section 2 Opener Image: Used with permission from Humenick SS. The clinical significance of breastmilk maturation rates. *Birth*. 1987;14:174-179.
Section 4 Opener Image: Adapted from Mott S. Nursing care of children and families. Redwood City, CA: Addison-Wesley; 1993:206.
Printing and Binding: Malloy, Inc.
Cover Printing: Malloy, Inc.

6048

Printed in the United States of America
15 14 13 12   10 9 8 7 6 5 4 3

DEDICATION

This book is dedicated to the memory of my mother, Martha Seem Hepp, who paid attention when her family doctor, Fred C. Rewerts, MD, said, "Aw, Martha, breastfeed 'em; they just do better," and went on to breastfeed three children in the late 1930s and early 1940s.

Contents

Suggestions for Using This Study Guide

This study guide, which accompanies the textbook *Breastfeeding and Human Lactation*, Fourth Edition, will help you assess your current knowledge of human lactation and prepare you for certification as a lactation consultant.

The study guide is organized to correspond with the fourth edition of the text published in 2009 by Jones and Bartlett Publishers. Every question (and its answer) in this study guide is linked with information in the fourth edition. Each chapter in this study guide contains the following:

- A list showing how information in that chapter applies to discipline areas tested on the certification examination offered by the International Board of Lactation Consultant Examiners (IBLCE).
- Multiple-choice questions that test the reader's understanding of facts about lactation and breastfeeding (answers are in the back of the book).
- Discussion questions that may or may not have a single best answer but are designed to spark discussion and prompt review of the topic addressed.

As compared with the previous edition of the study guide, this edition contains many more multiple-choice questions. These questions will better prepare you both for the IBLCE examination and for problems that you will encounter in clinical practice. More questions are posed on topics emphasized in the IBLCE exam. Either multiple-choice or discussion questions can be used to generate discussions in exam study groups, staff meetings, and journal clubs.

About the Questions in This Study Guide

Multiple-Choice Questions

Multiple-choice questions can sometimes be tedious to work through or tricky to interpret. Here are some tips to smooth the way:

- Each question begins with a stem—either a question or the beginning of a statement—followed by four options that answer the question or complete the statement.
- Each question has *one best* answer mixed in with the other options.
- In many cases, you will be able to quickly eliminate one or two obviously incorrect answers. Now you must ferret out the *one best* response from the remaining alternatives. These remaining alternatives are partly or entirely incorrect, or are correct but not the best alternative offered.

If you consistently pick correct answers, congratulations! If you don't, try to figure out what went wrong. Did you misread the question? Did you read only two or three of the possible answers, thereby selecting an alternative that was partially correct but not the one best answer? (Or, maybe you just didn't know the right response.) If you answered incorrectly, go back and reread the question and the correct answer. If you don't understand why a given answer is considered correct (or if you disagree with that answer), review the topic in the chapter of the same name in *Breastfeeding and Human Lactation*, Fourth Edition. More strategies are discussed at the end of this introductory material.

Discussion Questions

The discussion questions require you to organize what you understand about a topic into a coherent form, so that you can explain the topic—to yourself or to your colleagues. No answers are provided to these questions because your answers can rightfully be influenced by your own experiences as a lactation consultant as well as by information in the text.

Preparing for and Taking a Certification Exam

A certification examination tests two types of knowledge: what you know cognitively and how well you use that information when confronted with a problem. You can do best if you begin the test relaxed and ready to go—a state easier to achieve if you are well prepared.

The International Board of Lactation Consultant Examiners Examination

Most certification examinations, including the one administered by the International Board of Lactation Consultant Examiners, Inc. (IBLCE), consist of a long series of multiple-choice questions. Past IBLCE exams have contained about 200 questions. The certification examination is divided into morning and afternoon segments.

The morning session is devoted exclusively to multiple-choice questions. A test booklet contains all the information you need in order to answer each question; you can make notes in the booklet at will. You will record your answers on a separate machine-scorable answer sheet. On this answer sheet, be careful to mark the correct slot for a given question. Because your total score is based on the number of *correct* answers (not the number of wrong answers), make educated guesses even if you don't know the correct answer.

You will have about 3 hours to complete the morning session. You may leave the examination room when you are finished. If you finish early, review the questions you were unsure of. Even if you are a slow test taker, you should have sufficient time to complete the morning segment. However, if you

run out of time before you run out of questions, you will lose points. If you tend to take tests slowly, practice answering multiple-choice questions with four possible answers within a set time—no more than one minute per question—so that you can get a feel for how quickly you should proceed through the real examination.

During the afternoon session you will answer multiple-choice questions keyed to illustrations in a second test booklet. Practice for this portion beforehand by looking at slides or photographs of breastfeeding situations and then answering questions about them—questions that you make up or questions provided by the vendor of the illustrations.

Because the IBLCE seeks to determine minimum competency, you need not have the top score in order to be certified. Usually the lowest passing score is in the middle of the 60th percentile.

Before an Exam

Give yourself plenty of time to study—weeks or months rather than three all-nighters right before the exam. If you think of the exam as a performance, you can appreciate that regular, frequent rehearsals are the best preparation.

Many successful certification candidates meet with colleagues once or twice a week for several months; commonly, each assumes responsibility for leading a discussion about a particular topic. Then they go through study guide questions bearing on that chapter (or topic). Discussion questions can be used as a basis for writing additional multiple-choice questions—a good exercise that will nail down what you know and help you better analyze multiple-choice questions on exams.

The day before the exam, exercise vigorously enough so that you can relax and get a good night's sleep. Go to bed early; you will then be more alert and able to concentrate better on test day. On test-day morning, do yourself a favor: *Eat breakfast!* Taking a certification exam requires a lot of energy; you don't want to fade out midmorning. Your breakfast should contain enough protein and calories to keep you going for several hours and should sit lightly in your stomach. This isn't the time to try out a new recipe or to chow down so heavily that all you want to do is take a nap.

Staying Comfortable During an Exam

Sites

Examination sites differ. You may be asked to report to a hotel room, a college or hospital classroom, a church hall, or some other public meeting room not designed for test takers. Distracting noises may intrude into the room. Uneven lighting may make the exam hard to read or the illustrations difficult to see clearly. If such distractions are present, insist that your exam administrator make appropriate adjustments.

Clothing

Regardless of the season, it is best to dress in layers. Wear garments that you can easily take off or put back on. Bring a sweater—meeting rooms are generally chilly. Dress for comfort instead of style. Wear loose, casual clothing that you would choose for a daylong plane ride or car trip.

Snacks and Medicines

Physical discomfort, such as hunger, will distract you from the examination. If you are allowed to bring hard candies or other small snacks with you, do so. When you're struggling to think through a particularly knotty question, a bit of quick energy will help your performance. On the day of the exam, try to avoid taking medicines that make you drowsy.

Anxiety

If you begin to feel panicky during the exam, try one or more of these techniques:

- Take several deep breaths that expand your stomach. If you know breathing techniques for labor and childbirth, use them.
- Close your eyes and try to visualize yourself in a safe and relaxing place.
- Practice progressive relaxation by relaxing successive muscle groups. Begin with the tips of your toes and work up your body, or start at the top of your head and work down.
- If you feel your heart beating rapidly, tell yourself, "I'm going to breathe deeply, and my heart rate will slow." Then imagine your heart slowing as you breathe deeply and slowly several times.

- Some test takers say to themselves, "This is an easy exam," or "I know almost all of the answers," or "I know how to take this kind of exam." Such thoughts create a positive mindset.

No one has died from taking a certification exam. Enter the examination room alert to your surroundings and ready to concentrate on the task at hand. It is okay to feel a bit anxious—that feeling often will help give you a good "edge." Think of the exam questions as hurdles of differing heights, most of which you will easily sail over. Each time you answer a question, you've cleared a hurdle, and you will gain confidence in your ability to continue successfully.

Test-Taking Strategies

The following general strategies may help you move through an exam with confidence:

- Approach each question as if it were your only care in the world. Read it carefully all the way to the end.
- Concentrate on the question at hand. Don't read information into the question or allow your mind to wander back to previous questions.
- Eliminate clearly incorrect options before selecting from the remaining alternatives.
- Skip questions that stump you; come back to them at the end. By that time your mind is warmed up and the answer often will come easily.
- Trust your intuition; trust yourself. Your first hunch is usually right.
- Use the test booklet to jot down notes.
- Select the one option that you think is the best response.
- Record your answer correctly on the answer sheet.
- Once you've completed a question, put it out of your mind.

Some general comments about analyzing multiple-choice questions are discussed above. Now, let's talk about the IBLCE exam in particular.

- Words such as *always* and *never* will rarely be part of a correct answer.
- Look at the question stem first. The stem tells you what you need to look for (in the follow-

ing description or in an illustration) in order to pick the correct answer.

- Look for questions that ask for first (or last) actions—for example, "What would you do *first*?" Although all of the choices offered may describe correct actions, the one best answer will be the response that you will make first.

- Decide whether the stem is positive or negative before proceeding with the question. Note negative words and prefixes—for example, "All of the following are true *except*" or "*Not* breast-feeding is associated with . . ."

- For a question coupled with an illustration, first read the stem of the question. The stem will direct your attention to particular aspects of the illustration. Now look briefly at the illustration and get a sense of what you are looking at (or for). Then sort through the possible answers, always looking for that one best answer.

- Pace yourself. Try to complete each question within 1 minute. It is to your advantage to guess at remaining questions if you do not have time to analyze each of them.

Here are three examples of how to apply the techniques just described:

1. The most effective technique for using a textbook to study for an exam is to

   a. read the textbook as close to the exam date as possible.

   b. read the textbook a little at a time.

   c. write one or two questions that you think might be asked.

   d. concentrate on the summary information and the tables, if any.

   - Alternative a is clearly incorrect. Following its advice is likely to increase your anxiety and prevent you from getting through the material before the exam.

   - Alternative b is excellent advice, particularly when you are attempting to learn and remember a large body of information. It looks like it might be the one best answer—but don't stop here. Read all of the alternatives before you decide.

   - Alternative c is also good advice, but one or two questions are unlikely to be enough to

help you remember what you've read. This answer is partially correct, but not the one best answer.

   - Alternative d is good advice, but summary information and tables are unlikely to include some of the more detailed information that you may need to know. It is partially correct, but not the one best answer.

2. When confronted by a multiple-choice question you don't understand, you should

   a. select the most difficult-to-understand alternative.

   b. go back to the question later.

   c. select the one option you do understand.

   d. guess at the answer.

   - Alternative a is a poor choice. The less you understand, the less likely you are to select the correct answer.

   - Alternative b is a better choice. Time, relaxing a bit more, and getting into a test-taking mode may be all you need to understand the question more completely.

   - Alternative c may be the best choice. The option you understand is more likely than others to be the correct answer. Remember, the test writers are not trying to trick you. But don't stop here—read all of the alternatives before you decide on your answer.

   - Alternative d is a poor choice in practice if any other means are available. Improve your odds before guessing by eliminating any clearly incorrect alternatives. If you've reduced your choices to two then you have a 50:50 chance of guessing correctly. However, guessing from four options gives you only a 25 percent chance of correctly answering the question.

3. When you are taking a multiple-choice test that includes visual material, how should you approach the question?

   a. Look at the picture for at least 30 seconds, and then read the question.

   b. Read the stem of the question first, look at the photo, and then read the options.

   c. Read the stem of the question and all of the options; then look at the photo.

d. Look at the picture, and then read the options.

- Alternative a is a poor choice. Simply looking at the picture for a long period may not tell you what is being asked. You may lose valuable time following this advice.

- Alternative b is a good choice. By reading the stem of the question, you may obtain clues about what to look for in the visual material. These clues will help you select the correct option. But don't stop here—read all of the alternatives before deciding on your answer.

- Alternative c is a poor choice. If you spend too much time on the written portion of the question, you may not have enough time to examine the visual material.

- Alternative d is also a poor choice. The visual material may, in the absence of awareness of the stem, give you an incorrect impression when selecting the options.

The Exam Is Over!

When you've completed the examination, celebrate having survived—and then try to forget about it. It will be many weeks before you learn how well you did. Until the day you receive your certificate declaring that you are now a certified lactation consultant, concentrate on the rest of your busy and fulfilling life.

Additional Resources

New Online Interactive Testing Program

Enclosed within this study guide you will find a printed "access code card" containing an access code providing you access to the new online interactive testing program, JB TestPrep. This program will help you prepare for certification exams, such as the IBLCE's exam for becoming a certified lactation consultant. The online program includes the same multiple-choice questions that are printed in this study guide. You may sort the questions by chapter or randomize them. You can choose a "practice exam" that allows you to see feedback on your response immediately, or a "final exam," which hides your results until you have completed all the questions in the exam. Your overall score on the questions you have answered is also compiled. Here are the instructions on how to access JB TestPrep, the Online Interactive Testing Program:

1. Find the printed access code card bound in to this book.
2. Go to www.JBLearning.com/usecode.

3. Enter in your 10-digit access code, which you can find by scratching off the protective coating on the access code card.
4. Follow the instructions on each screen to set up your account profile and password. Please note: Only select a course coordinator if you have been instructed to do so by an institution or an instructor.
5. Contact Jones and Bartlett Publishers technical support if you have any questions:

   - Call 800-832-0034
   - Visit www.jbpub.com and select "Tech Support"
   - Email info@jbpub.com

Photo Library

The fourth edition of *Breastfeeding and Human Lactation* contains an electronic photo library that offers a number of photographs from the book on a CD-ROM. This photo library can help you prepare for the photo portion of the IBCLE exam.

Acknowledgments

I wish to recognize the efforts and astute comments of Anna Marie Heard, CMT(ASCP), and Mary Tagge, BSN, RN, IBCLC, who reviewed the multiple-choice questions in this study guide.

Mary-Margaret Coates

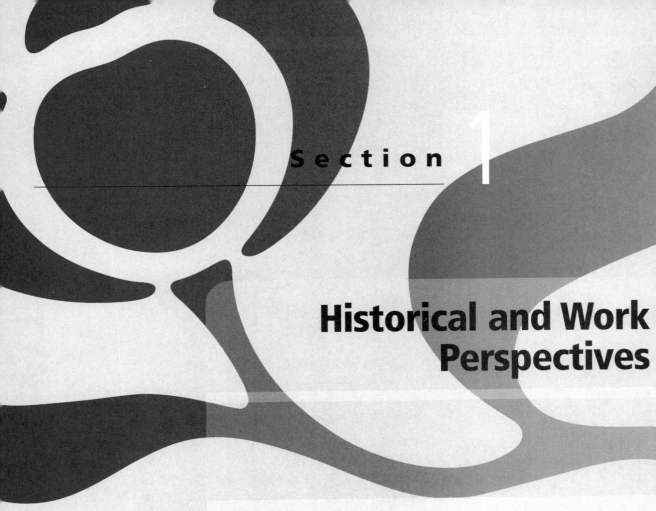

Section 1

Historical and Work Perspectives

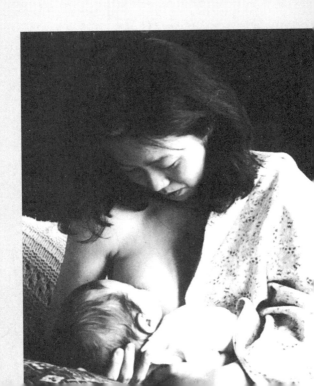

The Lactation Specialist: Roles and Responsibilities

Introduction

Lactation consultants are specialists who extend maternal–child health care in many settings. Questions in this chapter will help you assess your familiarity with practical ways that a lactation consultant can meet her professional and legal responsibilities to the mother and baby she is assisting, to her employer, and to society at large.

IBLCE Disciplines

Information in this chapter applies to the following disciplines tested on the certification examination offered by the International Board of Lactation Consultant Examiners: J = Ethical and Legal Issues; M = Public Health.

Multiple-Choice Questions

1. Most research studies of the effect of lactation consultant (LC) advice to a breastfeeding mother show that
   a. breastfeeding advice from LC-directed support groups does not increase the prevalence or duration of breastfeeding.
   b. face-to-face counseling increases initiation of exclusive breastfeeding but not total duration of breastfeeding.
   c. almost any contact between lactation consultants and new mothers increases the duration of breastfeeding.
   d. studies of rural populations show that lactation consultant advice may or may not promote breastfeeding, whereas studies of metropolitan populations show that it does.

2. A lactation consultant must record ("chart") each contact with a client. The information contained in these notes may do all of the following *except*

   a. be shared with others who care for the same client.

   b. be observations of the mother but not of the infant.

   c. demonstrate to insurers or in lawsuits that services were rendered.

   d. be incorporated into a research database.

3. In 2009, a clinical care plan for a new mother in hospital has all the following characteristics *except* that

   a. it provides basic information about assessment, diagnosis, and planned interventions.

   b. a standard plan for the patient's situation can be modified to fit the patient and may be handwritten.

   c. it is a requirement of the Joint Commission for hospital accreditation but not a legal requirement of practice.

   d. it is available to all caregivers who care for her.

4. The possibility of a lawsuit brought against a lactation consultant can be reduced by all of the following practices *except*

   a. approving of early discharge when a baby has not yet latched onto the breast.

   b. explaining what procedures you wish to perform and what information those procedures will elicit, and ask permission to proceed.

   c. keeping your knowledge of research findings up to date.

   d. documenting your assessment and interventions, and the rationale for them.

5. Lawsuits against healthcare workers may reflect a patient's anger because of

   a. a diagnosis that is incorrect.

   b. a treatment that is ineffective.

   c. records that are insufficiently detailed.

   d. a disrespectful attitude toward the patient.

6. Rules contained in the Health Insurance Portability and Accountability Act (HIPPA) of 1996 accomplish all of the following *except*

   a. standardize transfer of electronic health information between healthcare providers and health insurers.

   b. protect the privacy of those providing care to a given client.

   c. prevent a person's health information from being linked to that person.

   d. allow caregivers need-to-know access to a patient's health information.

7. To avoid plagiarism, whether you publish in a newsletter, peer-reviewed journal, or in-house guidelines, follow all of the following guidelines *except*

   a. credit permanent printed information, such as journal articles.

   b. short-lifetime materials, such as pamphlets or handouts, need not be credited.

   c. obtain permission before using any copyrighted material.

   d. cite information obtained from Web sites by its URL (uniform resource locator) address and date of access.

8. Lactation consultants are expected to practice in accordance with the WHO Code (International Code of Marketing of Breastmilk Substitutes). All of the following are prohibited by the code *except*

   a. accurate labels on infant formula containers.

   b. advertising of infant formula or bottles to the general public.

   c. providing formula samples to new mothers.

   d. providing gifts to healthcare providers.

9. As a lactation consultant, you see a mother and young breastfeeding infant for recent poor weight gain by the infant. You note that the infant is feverish and listless. What do you do now?

   a. Evaluate recent breastfeeding behavior, and suggest ways to stimulate the baby.

   b. Evaluate recent breastfeeding behavior, suggest ways to stimulate the baby, and offer suggestions on how to reduce fever in an infant.

   c. Evaluate recent breastfeeding behavior, suggest ways to stimulate the baby, offer suggestions on how to reduce fever in an infant, and mention the possibility that the baby should be seen by the family's healthcare provider.

   d. Refer the mother and baby to her family's healthcare provider; assure the mother that you will return to breastfeeding problems after the baby has been evaluated for medical problems.

10. A hospital with 3,000 deliveries a year, a 68 percent initiation of breastfeeding, and a newborn intensive care unit but no outpatient service should have approximately _____ full-time-equivalent lactation consultants.

    a. 3.5

    b. 4.5

    c. 5.5

    d. 6.5

11. Members of the International Board of Lactation Consultant Examiners' ethics and discipline committee are drawn from the

    a. board of directors of the International Board of Lactation Consultant Examiners.

    b. board of directors of the International Lactation Consultant Association.

    c. entire body of certified lactation consultants.

    d. entire membership of the International Lactation Consultant Association.

12. The duty to do good, be merciful, and care about others' well-being is called _____, a principle of ethics.

    a. autonomy

    b. beneficence

    c. ethical justice

    d. nonmaleficence

13. In the United States, a lactation consultant who is a licensed _____ can receive reimbursement as a healthcare provider.

    a. medical doctor (MD) only

    b. registered nurse (RN) only

    c. medical doctor, registered nurse, or certified nurse–midwife

    d. medical doctor, nurse practitioner, or physician assistant

Discussion Questions

1. Briefly distinguish the roles of a lactation consultant and a voluntary breastfeeding counselor.

2. Define assertiveness. Briefly note how assertiveness differs from aggressiveness as a means of reaching a goal or solving a problem.

3. List two advantages and two disadvantages of a solo lactation consultant practice as compared with a partnership or group practice.

4. Briefly discuss each of the following legal issues. Include in your discussion an example that clearly avoids the legal problem in question.
   • Touching the client
   • Offering a guarantee
   • Causing emotional distress
   • Confidentiality of information

5. Outline how in-hospital lactation consultants and private practice lactation consultants can work together to provide complete, long-term services to breastfeeding mothers in the community.

6. Which healthcare providers should work together to assist the mother of a breastfeeding baby who has failed to regain birth weight at 1 month of age? What information or skill can each provider best provide? How will the providers communicate with each other to provide optimal care in both the long and short term?

7. What are three sources of didactic or clinical breastfeeding education in your community that are available to persons who wish to sit the IBLCE exam?

8. Read the discussions of one 24-hour period on an Internet service pertaining to breastfeeding. (If you are not connected to such a service, seek help from a colleague who is.) What does review of these topics tell you about the concerns of lactation consultants today?

9. How do you respond if you are offered a contract to endorse a new nipple cream? Describe the rationale for your response.

Tides in Breastfeeding Practice

Introduction

This chapter tries to bridge some 70 million years of human history. On both an individual level (breast-feeding guidance) and a societal level (breastfeeding promotion) we aspire to achieve today what was the norm many generations ago. Questions in this chapter will help you to put into a longer perspective the historical basis for modern breastfeeding practices and the goals we hope to achieve.

IBLCE Disciplines

Information in this chapter applies to the following disciplines tested on the certification examination offered by the International Board of Lactation Consultant Examiners: I = Interpretation of Research; M = Public Health.

Multiple-Choice Questions

1. Breastfeeding research has been hindered by surveys typified by all of the following *except*

   a. age of infant when other liquid foods were added—not asked.

   b. age of infant when solid foods were added—not asked.

   c. lack of distinction between degrees of breastfeeding ("any" to "exclusive")—not asked.

   d. mothers' inability to adequately recall details of her course of breastfeeding.

2. Humans belong to a class of animals (Mammalia) whose principal distinguishing characteristic is

   a. breasts.

   b. forward-facing paired eyes.

   c. opposable thumbs.

   d. upright posture.

3. Which of the following patterns of breastfeeding is thought to have characterized humans before about 10,000 years ago?
    a. Feedings that were infrequent but long, day and night
    b. Frequent but brief breastfeeding bouts, day and night
    c. Infrequent daytime feedings, to accommodate mothers' work, coupled with frequent night feedings
    d. Total duration only until teeth erupted

4. It has been proposed that the natural age of complete weaning from the breast is 2–4 years of age, because in a young child
    a. lactose becomes a progressively larger part of the diet.
    b. molars have all erupted after about age 2 years, making it impossible to breastfeed without harming the mother.
    c. synthesis of lactase begins to decline about 2 years of age and is rare by 4 years of age.
    d. the "language explosion" during this age interval focuses the child on interaction with the entire family.

5. After weaning from the breast, a person's tolerance of lactose generally
    a. diminishes in societies that do not use animal milk as a food staple.
    b. increases in societies that use animal milk as a food staple.
    c. remains high in societies in which animal milk is not a food staple.
    d. remains unchanged in all known cultures.

6. Evidence shows that animal milk was first used as an infant food
    a. in the late 1800s, after the development of tinned milk in industrialized nations.
    b. less than 7,000 years ago, sometime after the development of animal husbandry.
    c. many millions of years ago—very early in human evolutionary history.
    d. only after wet-nursing fell out of favor as an alternative to maternal nursing.

7. Aid shipments of bovine milk from milk-consuming countries to countries that do not traditionally consume milk is a _____ idea, because bovine milk _____
    a. bad / is poorly digested by most recipients.
    b. bad / reduces local interest in food production.
    c. good / expands the variety of foods available to local peoples.
    d. good / stimulates a young child's immune system.

8. Hand-feeding foods other than breastmilk before a neonate is put to breast is practiced
    a. in both traditional and industrialized societies.
    b. only in highly traditional societies.
    c. principally on hospital-born infants in industrialized nations.
    d. rarely, owing to concern about the safety of such feedings.

9. Delay in putting an infant to breast combined with hand-feeding of a neonate is a set of practices that _____ undermines breastfeeding _____
   a. rarely / if the family and societal belief support subsequent breastfeeding.
   b. rarely / wherever they are practiced.
   c. typically / if promoted by the paternal grandmother.
   d. typically / wherever they are practiced.

10. On the basis of current practices of many traditional societies, long-term mixed feeding (at the breast plus hand-feeding of other fluids or soft solids) is
    a. indicated to accustom the infant to care from many people in the household.
    b. almost never practiced.
    c. common in the high latitudes, where bovine milk can be safely stored for a short time, but rare in more tropical countries.
    d. widely practiced in many societies.

11. Mixed feeding is common in the United States. In their first 3 months, infants were highly likely to be fed a mixed diet by mothers who share all of the following characteristics *except*
    a. aged 13–19 years old.
    b. formal education no higher than grade 12.
    c. married to a man not the baby's father.
    d. reside in a rural area.

12. Historically and at present, the factor most closely linked with infant mortality is
    a. a decline in the rate of any breastfeeding.
    b. a decline in the rate of exclusive breastfeeding.
    c. poverty.
    d. use of Western-style feeding patterns in non-Western settings.

13. Commercial advertising for manufactured infant milk typically plays upon all of the following themes *except*
    a. a mother's concern for her infant's well-being.
    b. difficulty of breastfeeding.
    c. lack of immunoglobulins in manufactured milks.
    d. nutritional similarity of the manufactured milk to breastmilk.

14. The most common reason given by a mother for feeding manufactured baby milk to her infant is
    a. baby awakens frequently at night.
    b. breastfeeding takes too much time.
    c. not enough breastmilk.
    d. sore nipples.

15. Feeding a young infant at fixed intervals
    a. accommodates variations in the infant's hunger only poorly.
    b. best ensures the infant's adequate nutrition.
    c. reduces crying in the infant.
    d. teaches the infant patience and self-control.

16. In the United States, the prevalence of breastfeeding dipped to its lowest point in the
    a. 1940s.
    b. 1960s.
    c. 1970s.
    d. early 1980s.

17. A decline in prevalence of breastfeeding that is associated with internal migration from rural to urban areas holds true in
    a. both developed and developing countries.
    b. developing nations only.
    c. those countries only that avoided being part of a colonial empire.
    d. the United States only during the interval of 1945–1970.

18. Infant mortality has tended to be highest—through time and around the world—in populations that are characterized by all of the following *except* they
    a. are very poor.
    b. breastfeed at high rates.
    c. breastfeed for long total durations.
    d. breastfeed at low rates.

19. A decline in breastfeeding prevalence may not be mirrored by an increase in infant mortality if
    a. infants are secluded in their families until they are about 3 years old.
    b. primary health care is widely available.
    c. the family diet contains sufficient protein and calories.
    d. the mother is able to read.

20. Surveys show that in the early 2000s, worldwide, about _____ percent of infants were fully or partially breastfed for at least 12 months.
    a. 45
    b. 60
    c. 85
    d. 95

21. The harmful effects of formula on infant health can be attributed *principally* to
    a. contamination of the product as it is prepared for feeding.
    b. feeding an amount of formula insufficient for the infant's needs.
    c. lack of immunological properties.
    d. presence of some constituents in nonphysiologic proportions.

22. As compared with a breastfeeding mother, a mother who does not breastfeed her infant is
    a. less likely to have osteoporosis develop, because calcium is not being removed from her system.
    b. less likely to have premenopausal breast cancer develop, because her hormonal status is more stable.
    c. more likely to develop diabetes, but not until later in life.
    d. removing a stressor on her body such that her long-term health will improve.

23. As compared with the cost of feeding formula, the cost of breastfeeding is _____ , in part because the _____
    a. higher / mother must consume high-quality foods in order to produce adequate breastmilk.
    b. higher / mother must seek medical care more frequently.
    c. lower / breastfed infant consumes less milk than a bottle-fed infant.
    d. lower / cost of manufactured milk is many times the cost of extra food for the mother who produces breastmilk.

24. As compared with infants fed formula, breastfed infants tend to have _____ illness, because _____
    a. less / breastmilk helps the infant resist bacterial infection.
    b. less / the protein in breastmilk is more concentrated.
    c. more / of the relatively dilute nature of human milk.
    d. more / the nutritional status of formula-fed infants is better.

25. Full breastfeeding promotes infant and child survival in all of the following ways *except*
    a. reducing exposure to dietary pathogens.
    b. increasing birth spacing of consecutive children, which increases the likelihood of survival of the younger but not older child.
    c. increasing birth spacing of consecutive children, which increases the likelihood of survival of both older and younger child.
    d. reducing the total number of children born into a family.

26. The Special Supplemental Nutrition Program for Women, Infants, and Children (the WIC program) is the United States' largest purchaser and distributor of infant formula. Even so, WIC reaches out to breastfeeding women by allowing them all of the following *except*
    a. longer benefits—1 year.
    b. more, and more varied, food supplements.
    c. no access to free infant formula.
    d. priority for enrollment in WIC programs.

27. Mothers enrolled in WIC initiate breastfeeding at a rate that is
    a. comparable to the rate of mothers at large.
    b. higher than mothers of a heritage (such as Hispanic or Asian) in which breastfeeding is common.
    c. lower than mothers who qualify for WIC enrollment but who did not enroll.
    d. much higher than the rate of mothers at large.

28. In the United States, a mother's legal right to breastfeed in public is protected by all of the following *except*
    a. federal law that permits her to breastfeed in all public gathering places.
    b. federal law that permits her to breastfeed in any place she is entitled to be.
    c. law in some states that prevents charges of indecent exposure.
    d. law in some states that permits her to breastfeed in any place she is entitled to be.

29. The International Code of Marketing of Breast-Milk Substitutes
    a. allows public advertising of infant formula.
    b. forbids, while a mother and baby are in a health institution, the mother's use of infant formula.
    c. forbids distribution of free infant formula samples directly to mothers.
    d. supports distribution of breastfeeding information by infant formula manufacturers.

30. The principles of the Baby-Friendly Hospital Initiative require that health facilities providing maternity services do all of the following *except*
    a. allow mothers and infants to remain together 24 hours a day.
    b. encourage breastfeeding on demand.
    c. give newborn infants nothing by mouth other than breastmilk—except sterile water—unless medically indicated.
    d. help mothers initiate breastfeeding within 30 minutes after birth.

31. By far the largest number of baby-friendly hospitals are in
    a. developed nations, where needed technology is available.
    b. developed nations, whose move to act on baby-friendly principles is only weakly opposed by infant milk manufacturers.
    c. developing nations, because fewer staff are available to care for the mother–infant dyad.
    d. developing nations, in part because adherence to the baby-friendly program can be mandated by the government.

32. As compared with women who give birth elsewhere, women who give birth in a baby-friendly hospital are
    a. less likely to initiate breastfeeding, but those who do continue longer.
    b. more likely to both initiate breastfeeding and to continue for a longer time.
    c. more likely to initiate breastfeeding, but no more likely to continue.
    d. no more likely to initiate breastfeeding.

D i s c u s s i o n   Q u e s t i o n s

1. What constitute normal breastfeeding practices?

2. What is wet-nursing? Why is it rarely practiced in industrialized countries today?

3. What is hand-feeding?

4. Name three hand-fed foods. Describe their effect on the nutritional status and general health of a 1-month-old infant and on a 6-month-old infant.

5. What are prelacteal feeds? Offer at least three explanations for their use in various cultures or time periods.

6. How do you explain the relationship in many parts of the world between high breastfeeding rates and high infant mortality?

7. Identify and briefly discuss four health risks resulting from the use of manufactured baby milks. Explain why some health risks appear to be short term, whereas others are long term.

8. Briefly describe three aspects of cost incurred by feeding manufactured milks to infants ("cost" may be considered in financial or in other terms).

   • Cost to a family

   • Cost to the family's community

   • Cost to the broader society

9. What is the WHO Code? Why is it important in a developing country? Why is it important in a developed country?

10. Describe the ten steps of the Baby-Friendly Hospital Initiative.

11. Explain the role of advertising in increasing the use of manufactured baby milks. Give three examples of how these products are advertised to the public and to healthcare professionals.

12. Identify how class differences in both an industrialized country and a non-industrialized country have influenced the likelihood of breastfeeding initiation and its duration. If the patterns of behavior are different, how do you explain this difference?

13. What is "breastfeeding promotion"? How does it differ from "breastfeeding support"? Outline three ways in which breastfeeding might be promoted.

14. Explain why both the older and the younger infant are at greater risk of death when birth spacing is short.

15. Price the cost of 150 cans of ready-to-feed manufactured baby milk, about the number of cans used during a baby's first 6 months. What proportion of income must be assigned to the purchase of manufactured infant milk by a family whose monthly income is

    • $500?

    • $1,000?

    • $2,500?

16. Exclusive feeding of manufactured milk is likely to lead to what other expenditures? Estimate the cost of those other expenditures.

17. How would you implement each of the Ten Steps to Successful Breastfeeding in a healthcare facility in your community? Which steps would you implement first? Why? How would you ensure that each step is implemented?

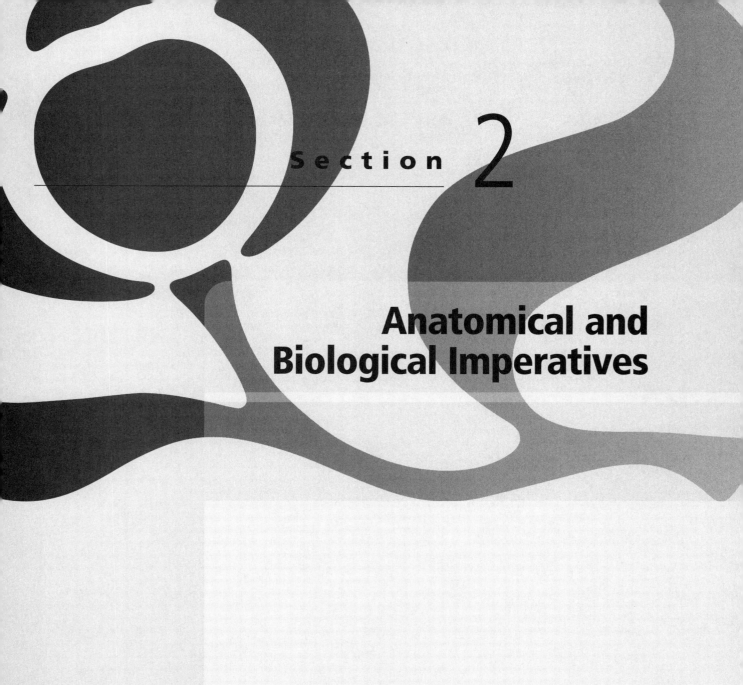

Section 2

Anatomical and Biological Imperatives

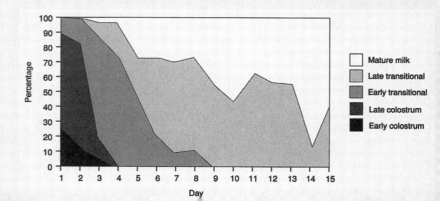

Anatomy and
Physiology of Lactation

Introduction

Everything we do as lactation consultants is influenced by our understanding of the anatomy of the human breast, the physiology of milk production, the mechanisms of infant suckling, and the responses that drive infant suckling. We must be well grounded in this material before we can thoroughly assess a breastfeeding dyad. Questions in this chapter will help you to assess your understanding of this body of essential information and how it applies to professional practice.

IBLCE Disciplines

Information in this chapter applies to the following disciplines tested on the certification examination offered by the International Board of Lactation Consultant Examiners: A = Maternal and Infant Anatomy; E = Maternal and Infant Pathology; H = Growth Parameters, and Developmental Milestones; L = Techniques; 4 = Prematurity; 12 = General Principles.

Multiple-Choice Questions

1. The breasts begin to develop by the fourth week of gestation, and by the fifth week a region of thickened epithelial cells develops that is limited to

   a. the areas immediately underlying the areas that will become the breasts.

   b. two lines that extend from the scapula (shoulder blade) to the groin.

   c. two lines that extend from the axilla (armpit) to the groin.

   d. two lines that extend from the axilla (armpit) to the area underlying the breasts.

2. After birth, the newborn's mammary tissue may secrete a
   a. colostrum-like fluid in both male and female infants.
   b. colostrum-like fluid in female but not in male infants.
   c. plasma-like fluid in male but not in female infants.
   d. plasma-like fluid in both male and female infants.

3. After about 12 years of age in girls, breast structures display all activities listed below *except* that
   a. buds form on ducts ends; the buds will become alveoli in the mature breast.
   b. during each subsequent cycle, ductal extension continues from a somewhat regressed position.
   c. during ovulatory menstrual cycles, estrogen fosters mammary development.
   d. primary and secondary ducts divide and extend during each menstrual cycle.

4. Breast structures complete their functional development
   a. after about age 27.
   b. during pregnancy.
   c. during the first 72 hours postpartum.
   d. mediated by release of estrogen during sexual intercourse.

5. The milk-forming unit of the breast is composed of all of the following *except*
   a. a double layer of epithelial cells in which milk is formed.
   b. an alveolar lumina in which droplets collect.
   c. ductules that merge with ducts.
   d. myoepithelial cells that contract and eject milk into ductules.

6. Milk ducts, as they travel between the point at which several ductules join and the nipple pores, follow which kind of path?
   a. Meandering, and crossing and recrossing other ducts
   b. Meandering, but without impinging on other ducts
   c. Relatively straight and at a slight angle to each other as they converge on the nipple
   d. Relatively straight and parallel, in a central cluster

7. Which of the following statements is true?
   a. Each normal breast contains at least 20 lobes containing alveoli, ductules, and ducts.
   b. Infants should take a big "mouthful" of areola in order to obtain milk that pools in sinuses in milk ducts under the areola.
   c. Lobes do not interconnect with each other, except for some ducts that merge near the nipple.
   d. The milk-secreting alveolus is constructed of a single layer of epithelial cells.

8. Milk is secreted in alveoli, where it remains until a signal from the hormone _____, produced by the _____ gland, causes _____ cells to contract and force milk into milk ductules.
   a. oxytocin / anterior pituitary / squamous cuboidal
   b. oxytocin / posterior pituitary / myoepithelial
   c. prolactin / anterior pituitary / squamous cuboidal
   d. prolactin / posterior pituitary / myoepithelial

9. The amount of adipose tissue in the breast is _____ related to _____.

    a. directly / the mother's milk-producing capacity.

    b. directly / the mother's milk-storage capacity.

    c. inversely / the mother's milk-storage capacity.

    d. not / either milk-production or milk-storage capacity.

10. For at least the first 6 months of lactation, the average normal adult breast typically

    a. about doubles in weight.

    b. increases in weight by half.

    c. steadily gains weight as infant intake increases.

    d. steadily loses weight as fat tissue is metabolized.

11. A structure that attaches deep breast tissue to the skin is called a(an)

    a. axillary tail.

    b. Cooper's ligament.

    c. Montgomery's tubercle.

    d. pectoralis majora.

12. Blood is delivered to the breast principally by which artery or arteries?

    a. Axillary

    b. Internal mammary

    c. Lateral thoracic

    d. Subclavian

    e. Only a and b

    f. Only b and c

13. The number of ducts that produce openings in the nipple ("nipple pores") is usually

    a. about 4.

    b. about 9.

    c. about 12.

    d. the same number as the number of lobes in the breast.

14. Milk ducts have all of the following characteristics *except* that they are not

    a. deep seated.

    b. easily compressed.

    c. known to vary in diameter.

    d. small.

15. A lateral incision at which position listed below is most likely to sever the nerve that innervates the nipple and areola? Right and left refer to the mother's right and left sides.

    a. 5 o'clock on the right, 7 o'clock on the left

    b. 7 o'clock on the right, 5 o'clock on the left

    c. 8 o'clock on the right, 4 o'clock on the left

    d. 9 o'clock on the right, 3 o'clock on the left

16. Nipple diameter that greatly exceeds the average diameter of about 16 mm is reported to be associated with
    a. early infant weight gain greater than 1 ounce per day.
    b. infant choking during initial, but not subsequent, letdown.
    c. infant colic related to excess intake of foremilk.
    d. infant difficulty latching on.

17. All of the following statements about areolar glands are true *except* that they
    a. are most abundant on the areola but also are found elsewhere on the breast.
    b. combine milk and sebaceous glands.
    c. are more apt to be located on the upper, lateral side of the areola.
    d. are directly associated with rapid infant weight gain.

18. Which of the following statements about breast symmetry is true?
    a. Breasts are almost always of the same size (symmetrical).
    b. When breasts are asymmetrical, the right breast usually is larger than the left.
    c. Asymmetry usually reflects a difference in the number of lobes rather than a difference in size of lobes.
    d. An extremely small, narrow breast may be a marker for problems producing milk.

19. Accessory nipples and underlying breast tissue
    a. rarely occur except in the groin.
    b. may swell slightly at the time of lactogenesis II but do not produce milk.
    c. may occur anywhere along the primitive milk line.
    d. almost always develop in pairs.

20. Which statement about nipple protractility (eversion of the nipple by gentle compression of the base of the nipple) during pregnancy is *false*?
    a. Nipples tend to be less protractile during a first pregnancy than during subsequent pregnancies.
    b. The degree of nipple protactility increases during a given pregnancy.
    c. About 10–35 percent of women show poor nipple protractility during their first pregnancy.
    d. Poor nipple protractility is closely related to breastfeeding difficulty.

21. During pregnancy, the nipple grows under the influence of _____ and the areola under the influence of _____ in maternal serum.
    a. estrogen / prolactin
    b. placental lactogen / estrogen
    c. progesterone / prolactin
    d. prolactin / placental lactogen

22. During pregnancy, mammary ducts proliferate under the influence of _____, and mammary lobes grow under the influence of _____ in maternal serum.
    a. estrogen / progesterone
    b. placental lactogen / estrogen
    c. progesterone / estrogen
    d. progesterone / placental lactogen

23. After a minimum of _____ weeks of pregnancy, a woman's body will produce milk even if the pregnancy ends at that time.
    a. 12
    b. 16
    c. 20
    d. 24

24. Lactogenesis I is correctly characterized by which of the following statements?
    a. Breast size increases because milk secretory cells swell with water.
    b. Epithelial cells differentiate into milk secretory cells.
    c. In a normal pregnancy it is complete by month 6.
    d. Tight junctions form between secretory cells.

25. Which of the following statements is *false*? Lactogenesis II will typically occur
    a. even if breasts are not stimulated by a nursing baby or by a pump in the first two or three days postpartum.
    b. later in women who have insulin-dependent diabetes.
    c. only if fluid is actually removed from the breasts by a nursing baby or by a pump in the first two or three days postpartum.
    d. sooner if breasts are stimulated by a nursing baby or by a pump in the first two or three days postpartum.

26. Lactogenesis II is correctly characterized by all of the following statements *except*
    a. by postpartum day 8, control of milk production switches from autocrine to endocrine.
    b. copious milk secretion begins, typically, on postpartum day 3.
    c. maternal progesterone concentration drops rapidly.
    d. tight junctions in the alveolar cell close.

27. After the placenta is delivered, _____ decrease, while _____ increase.
    a. milk fat and lactose / sodium and protein
    b. protein and lactose / sodium and milk fat
    c. sodium and milk fat / protein and lactose
    d. sodium and protein / milk fat and lactose

28. After the placenta is delivered, which of the following changes in hormone concentration takes place? Concentration(s) of progesterone
    a. and prolactin fall, but concentration of oxytocin rises.
    b. falls, but concentration of oxytocin and prolactin rise.
    c. prolactin and oxytocin all rise.
    d. remains stable, but concentrations of prolactin and oxytocin rise.

29. Prolactin is released from the
    a. anterior pituitary.
    b. hypothalamus.
    c. posterior pituitary.
    d. thyroid.

30. Galactopoiesis refers to the
    a. long-term maintenance of milk synthesis.
    b. maintenance of milk supply after supplementary foods are added to baby's diet.
    c. periodic upward adjustment of milk supply to match baby's increased demand.
    d. postengorgement downward adjustment of milk supply to match baby's demand.

31. Which of the following statements about breast involution is correct?
    a. Alveoli are removed and replaced by highly vascular connective tissue.
    b. Involution begins on average 21 days after the addition of supplements or the final breastfeeding.
    c. Involution is triggered by high concentrations of inhibitory peptides.
    d. Milk from an involuting breast contains low concentrations of sodium.

32. Which statement below is *not* correct?
    a. Progesterone can inhibit lactation postpartum if placental fragments are retained.
    b. Progesterone concentration reestablishes itself at about one half of its pregnancy concentration by four days after childbirth.
    c. Progesterone in high concentration maintains pregnancy.
    d. Progesterone inhibits lactation during pregnancy.

33. Once lactation is initiated, the principle hormone maintaining milk production is
    a. dopamine.
    b. insulin.
    c. oxytocin.
    d. prolactin.

34. Prolactin concentration in maternal blood
    a. attains highest values at the time that milk composition changes to mature milk.
    b. increases directly with the frequency and intensity (but not duration) of nipple stimulation.
    c. normally doubles in response to suckling.
    d. peaks about 90 minutes after the beginning of a breastfeeding bout.

35. In a mother who does not breastfeed, prolactin concentration usually returns to its nonpregnant value by _____ week(s) postpartum.
    a. 1
    b. 2
    c. 3
    d. 6

36. All of the following statements about the serum concentration of prolactin during established lactation are true *except*
    a. higher prolactin concentration delays the return of ovulation.
    b. prolactin concentration is closely related to milk yield.
    c. prolactin concentration is higher at night than in the day.
    d. prolactin concentration rises shortly after suckling begins at each feeding.

37. Which of the following statements is *not* correct? Prolactin concentrations are

    a. directly related to the degree of postpartum engorgement.

    b. elevated in response to anxiety or psychological stress.

    c. reduced in response to depression.

    d. reduced in women who smoke cigarettes.

38. Following birth, how is serum prolactin concentration affected by suckling? Assume 10 to 12 feedings per 24-hour day.

    a. It peaks with each suckling episode and declines markedly between feeds.

    b. It peaks with each suckling episode and remains near peak concentrations between feeds.

    c. It gradually drops to baseline during the first few weeks and remains there during the course of breastfeeding.

    d. It gradually climbs during the first few weeks of breastfeeding and then plateaus.

39. Which statement below is *not* correct? Normal prolactin concentration

    a. is 20 ng/ml or less in nonpregnant, nonlactating women.

    b. peaks at about 90 ng/ml in breastfeeding women at 10 days postpartum.

    c. declines slowly from peak concentration until, at about 6 months postpartum, it returns to prepregnant concentration.

    d. is higher in breastfeeding women whose menses have not returned than in women who are menstruating.

40. Maternal concentrations of prolactin differ in time and compartment. Which response is correct? Maternal concentration of prolactin is higher in

    a. hindmilk than in foremilk.

    b. mature milk than in early transitional milk.

    c. milk (average concentration) than in maternal plasma.

    d. Only a and b.

    e. Only a and c.

41. During the first few days postpartum, frequent suckling should be encouraged for all the reasons listed below *except* that frequent suckling

    a. is needed to initiate lactogenesis II.

    b. may increase the number of prolactin receptors in the breast.

    c. stimulates the milk letdown reflex.

    d. stimulates uterine contractions

42. Which statement is *not* correct? Prolactin-inhibiting factor

    a. can be suppressed by drugs such as metoclopramide.

    b. can be suppressed by nipple stimulation.

    c. stimulates the release of dopamine.

    d. stimulates the secretion of milk.

43. Oxytocin is released from the
    a. anterior pituitary.
    b. hypothalamus.
    c. posterior pituitary.
    d. thyroid.

44. Which of the following statements is *not* correct?
    a. Oxytocin causes myoepithelial cells to contract and propel milk into ductules.
    b. Oxytocin ceases release about 1 minute after cessation of nipple stimulation.
    c. Oxytocin is released in discrete pulses.
    d. Oxytocin is released into the mother's bloodstream within 1 minute after the beginning of suckling.

45. All of the following are secondary effects of oxytocin release into maternal blood *except*
    a. a heightened maternal calmness.
    b. a slight drop in maternal breast temperature.
    c. continued milk production.
    d. uterine contractions.

46. Increased skin temperature during a breastfeeding episode is produced by the release into the maternal bloodstream of
    a. cortisol.
    b. oxytocin.
    c. prolactin.
    d. thyroid-stimulating hormone.

47. As compared with a mother who exclusively breastfeeds her young infant, a mother who supplements her infant with formula will experience
    a. higher plasma concentration of oxytocin and prolactin.
    b. higher plasma concentration of oxytocin but lower concentration of prolactin.
    c. lower plasma concentration of oxytocin and prolactin.
    d. lower plasma concentration of prolactin but higher concentration of oxytocin.

48. The rate at which the breast synthesizes milk
    a. decreases as the length of time since the previous breastfeed increases.
    b. decreases from first morning feed through the rest of the day.
    c. increases as the age of the infant increases.
    d. increases as the amount of milk in the breast increases.

49. To synthesize milk, the mammary secretory cells obtain nutrients directly from the maternal bloodstream, which in turn obtains nutrients from the mother's
    a. current food intake.
    b. extracellular spaces near the alveoli.
    c. fat stores.
    d. liver.

50. In the first 3 days postpartum, the amount of colostrum secreted is
    a. directly related to the gestational age of the newborn.
    b. greater in breastfeeding women than in nonbreastfeeding women.
    c. greater in heavier women than in slimmer women.
    d. similar in breastfeeding women and nonbreastfeeding women.

51. The daily volume of milk that a given mother produces usually depends upon all of the following *except* how
    a. energetically her infant suckles.
    b. frequently her baby suckles.
    c. large is the mother's innate capacity for producing milk.
    d. much milk the baby takes per day.

52. Which of the following statements is *not* true? Women who experience galactorrhea
    a. can express some milk or serous fluid from their breasts long after ceasing to breastfeed.
    b. may have a pituitary tumor.
    c. may have begun use of certain intrauterine contraceptive devices.
    d. typically have prolactin concentrations more than double normal baseline concentration.

53. Adequately functioning breast tissue is generally indicated by all of the following *except*
    a. a wide flat space between the breasts.
    b. breast tenderness.
    c. increase in breast size.
    d. swelling of the breasts in the early postpartum.

54. Breast reduction surgery is most likely to
    a. have no effect on maternal milk production.
    b. increase milk production because of removal of fat tissue pinching milk ducts.
    c. reduce milk production because adipose tissue is disrupted.
    d. reduce milk production because nerves to the nipple are severed.

55. Thickening or dimpling of skin on the breast may be a sign of a
    a. brassiere that is rubbing.
    b. cancerous breast tumor.
    c. particularly robust milk-producing lobe.
    d. topical allergic reaction.

56. Second- and third-degree burns to the chest typically reduce all of the following *except*
    a. elasticity of the nipple.
    b. milk amount ejected at each suckle.
    c. sensation in the nipple.
    d. volume of glandular tissue to any significant degree.

57. Recent studies find that suckling behavior develops
    a. after birth in premature infants born between 28 and 32 weeks.
    b. before swallowing behavior.
    c. early in gestation—by 24 weeks.
    d. late in gestation—after 32 weeks.

58. The newborn's tongue occupies what percentage of its oral cavity?
    a. About a quarter
    b. About a half
    c. About 80 percent
    d. Nearly all

59. Which of the following responses is *not* correct? At birth, the infant's hard palate
    a. contains transverse ridges.
    b. is similar to that of an adult.
    c. is wide and only slightly arched.
    d. works with the tongue to hold and compress the nipple.

60. In the extraction of milk by the infant, vacuum in the infant's mouth plays a
    a. major role, likely, in milk removal.
    b. major role, occasionally, when the infant's oral cavity is small.
    c. small role, occasionally, when the infant's oral cavity is large.
    d. small role, usually, in milk removal.

61. A healthy infant who has difficulty properly latching onto and milking the breast is most likely to have which of the following conditions?
    a. A frenulum that is too long or too far back on the tongue
    b. A frenulum that is too short or too far forward under the tongue
    c. Buccal fat pads that are too thick and impinge upon the tongue
    d. Buccal fat pads that are too thin and do not support the cheeks

62. Which of the following responses is *not* true? Babies' rate of suckle and swallow
    a. is about once per second when milk is flowing.
    b. increases when milk flow decreases.
    c. increases when milk flow increases.
    d. maintains a more or less uniform rate during a breastfeeding bout.

63. Active suckling, in addition to providing milk for the infant, also decreases all of the following in the mother *except*
    a. feelings of anxiety.
    b. heart rate.
    c. metabolic rate.
    d. pain threshold.

64. Attempting to force a crying baby to latch onto the breast is likely to cause the baby to
    a. consider the breast to be a "pacifier."
    b. initiate rooting behavior.
    c. place its tongue against its hard palate.
    d. tear a tight frenulum.

65. Nonnutritive suckling by premature infants promotes which of the following?
    a. Decreased crying
    b. Increased gastrointestinal peristalsis
    c. Increased secretion of digestive fluids
    d. Only a and c
    e. Only a, b, and c

66. A newborn will increase suckling activity in response to a
    a. bitter taste.
    b. salt taste.
    c. sour taste.
    d. sweet taste.

67. How does a neonate's tongue move with normal suckling at the breast?
    a. From side to side as tongue is extended
    b. In a peristaltic motion from back to front
    c. In a peristaltic motion from front to back
    d. In a peristaltic motion solely up and down

68. As compared with an infant who is bottle fed, a baby fed at the breast
    a. feeds about the same number of times per 24-hour day.
    b. has a larger requirement for water.
    c. has a lower skin temperature.
    d. maintains a higher level of oxygen in his blood.

69. Cyanosis during a feeding
    a. is common only in neonates who have other medical problems.
    b. in neonates is typically followed by spontaneous recovery.
    c. is more common in older infants than in neonates.
    d. is rare, regardless of feeding method.

70. A newborn typically breathes through the
    a. mouth, because fewer breaths are needed to obtain a given volume of air.
    b. mouth, because the flat, flared nares restrict air flow.
    c. nose, because inhaled air is thus warmed before it travels to the lungs.
    d. nose, because of the relative volumes of the oral cavity and the tongue.

71. Normal, well-coordinated suckling, swallowing, and breathing follow a pattern such that
    a. a breath usually follows every one or two suck-swallows.
    b. breaths typically vary in depth—some are deep; others are shallow.
    c. pauses between clusters of suck-swallows are about the same length.
    d. suck-swallows cluster, and breaths are taken only in pauses between the clusters.

Discussion Questions

1. Discuss the relation between breast size and function in terms of lactational capacity.

2. Describe the form, location, and function in lactation of each of the following structures:
   • Lactiferous duct
   • Adipose cells
   • Milk glands
   • Myoepithelial cells
   • Nipple
   • Areola

3. Explain the relation between prolactin release, oxytocin release, milk production, and milk ejection.

4. Distinguish between breastfeeding and bottle-feeding in terms of the following:
   • Infant sounds while feeding
   • Frequency of feeding
   • Breathing patterns
   • Mouth extension
   • Tongue placement and action
   • Lip shape and position
   • Feeding duration

5. "What the baby does is a simple activity, involving negative pressure and swallowing what he or she obtains." Does this statement jibe with current thought? Why or why not?

6. What is meant by the supply-and-demand response of the lactating breast?

7. Explain the relationship between breast size, milk production, and milk storage capacity.

8. Outline a short presentation to a prenatal class on the following topics:
   • How the breast produces milk
   • The baby's contribution to successful breastfeeding

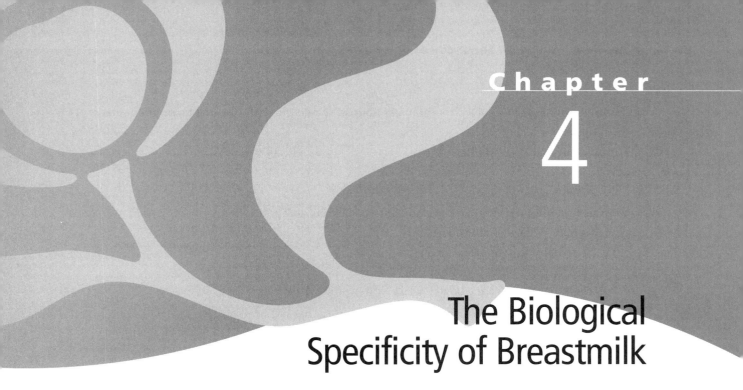

The Biological Specificity of Breastmilk

Introduction

During the long course of mammalian evolution, the milk of each species has acquired properties that meet the nutritional, immunological, and developmental needs of the infants for whom it is, for some period of time, the sole nutriment. Because the physical and cognitive abilities of neonates of different species differ widely (consider, for instance, newborn whales, mice, musk ox, and humans), so do the constituents of mothers' milk. A thoughtful lactation consultant must understand the basic biology of human milk and how it influences breastfeeding practices. Questions in this chapter will help you assess your knowledge of this essential body of information and how it applies to professional practice.

IBLCE Disciplines

Information in this chapter applies to the following disciplines tested on the certification examination offered by the International Board of Lactation Consultant Examiners: B = Maternal and Infant Normal Physiology and Endocrinology; C = Maternal and Infant Normal Nutrition and Biochemistry; H = Growth Parameters and Developmental Milestones; G = Psychology, Sociology, and Anthropology; I = Interpretation of Research; 4 = Prematurity; 5 = 0–2 days; 12 = General Principles.

Multiple-Choice Questions

1. Breastmilk is sometimes referred to as "white blood" because it can do all of the following *except*
   a. affect biochemical systems.
   b. deliver oxygen.
   c. destroy pathogens.
   d. transport nutrients.

2. Animal milks have evolved to optimally nourish the young within which taxonomic category?

    a. Class

    b. Family

    c. Order

    d. Species

3. Which of the following does *not* influence breastmilk composition?

    a. Gestational age of a newborn

    b. Maternal intake of fat-soluble vitamins

    c. Overall duration of lactation

    d. The point during a feeding at which composition is measured

4. A healthy mother in whom copious milk production has not been observed 3 days (72 hours) after an uneventful labor and delivery of a healthy baby

    a. is a cause for concern but is within the normal range of time at which this event occurs.

    b. is probably experiencing an effect of unrecognized gestational diabetes.

    c. should be evaluated for endocrine problems that might inhibit lactogenesis II.

    d. should have her baby's suck evaluated for effectiveness.

5. Compared with mature milk, colostrum is richer in

    a. carbohydrates but lower in protein.

    b. fats but lower in protein and minerals.

    c. protein and minerals but lower in carbohydrates and fats.

    d. protein but lower in minerals and carbohydrates.

6. The total daily dose of immunoglobulins received by a breastfed infant

    a. decreases as milk volumes increase, because the increased volume largely reflects additional water.

    b. increases as milk volumes increase, because older infants take more hind milk, where immunoglobulins reside.

    c. increases as milk volumes increase, because the infant takes greater volumes overall.

    d. remains more or less constant, even though the increased volume largely reflects additional water.

7. What is the approximate proportion of water to other components in human milk?

    a. 90:10

    b. 80:20

    c. 70:30

    d. 60:40

8. As compared with the average time required by formula, the average time in which about half of a meal of breastmilk empties from an infant's stomach is

    a. a little bit shorter.

    b. about the same.

    c. much shorter.

    d. typically slightly longer.

9. Healthy, growing, exclusively breastfed infants need water in addition to breastmilk if they

   a. are premature.

   b. live in a hot, dry climate.

   c. live in a hot, humid climate.

   d. None of the above.

10. The approximate calorie content of human milk is _____ per deciliter.

   a. 48

   b. 65

   c. 78

   d. 85

11. The American Academy of Pediatrics recommends that the calorie content of artificial infant milks be 67 kilocalories per deciliter. Why is that? As compared with breastfed infants, formula-fed infants need a food with a _____ calorie content, _____.

   a. quite a bit higher / because they do not digest formula well.

   b. quite a bit higher / to make up for smaller volumes ingested because they also take supplemental water.

   c. lower / in order to avoid overfeeding, because they tend to be less active.

   d. similar / so formula has a calorie content similar to that of breastmilk.

12. During their first four months, healthy, fully breastfed infants ingest nutrient intakes that are about _____ current (traditional) recommendations.

   a. 10 percent greater than

   b. 10 percent less than

   c. 20 percent less than

   d. the same as

13. As an exclusively breastfed baby grows, the energy value (kilocalories) of breastmilk ingested per kilogram of body weight changes how in the first few months?

   a. Decreases by about half

   b. Decreases by less than 30 percent

   c. Increases a little

   d. Increases by about 20 percent

14. As compared with infants bottle-fed manufactured milk, breastfed infants have lower average measured values in all of the following *except*

   a. heart rate.

   b. oxygenation.

   c. rectal temperature.

   d. total daily energy expenditure.

15. The breast produces a small amount of colostrum during the first 24 hours postpartum. In round numbers, how much is that?

    a. Average, about 100 ml (range, about 40–140 ml)

    b. Average, about 70 ml (range, about 40–140 ml)

    c. Average, about 40 ml (range, about 10–120 ml)

    d. Average, about 20 ml (range, about 5–100 ml)

16. The mother of a fully breastfed infant produces an average volume of breastmilk on day 5 postpartum of _____ ml per day, and at 6 months postpartum an average volume of _____ ml per day.

    a. 200 / 400

    b. 300 / 1,200

    c. 400 / 1,200

    d. 500 / 800

17. In thriving, exclusively breastfed infants, the total daily amount of breastmilk ingested during 1 month through 4 months of age increases

    a. gradually (by only 100 ml or so) as infant metabolism becomes more efficient.

    b. in stepwise fashion after growth spurts at 6 weeks and 3 months.

    c. not at all, as the fat (and thus calorie) content of milk increases.

    d. steadily (by 200–300 ml) as the infant's weight doubles.

18. As compared with first-time mothers at 1 week postpartum, multiparous mothers (those who have given birth before) at 1 week postpartum produce about _____ milk.

    a. 10 percent less

    b. 5 percent more

    c. 20 percent more

    d. the same amount of

19. As compared with the breastmilk produced by women in their 30s, the milk produced by adolescent mothers

    a. contains fewer calories, because fat content is lower.

    b. contains more protein, because more protein circulates in mothers whose immune system is still maturing.

    c. is about the same.

    d. typically is of smaller volume.

20. The ability of the breast to synthesize milk typically

    a. exceeds the infant's demand throughout the course of lactation.

    b. falls below the infant's needs by about 4 months.

    c. meets the infant's need with little to spare, in order to conserve maternal energy.

    d. proceeds at about the same rate in each breast.

21. Milk output generally is _____ from the _____ breast, probably because _____.

    a. larger / left / the baby tends to be cradled in the left arm.

    b. larger / right / it receives the greater flow of blood.

    c. smaller / left / the baby nurses more fitfully in order to keep his right eye free.

    d. smaller / right / it is offered to the infant fewer times per day.

22. Which statement below is *not* true? As compared with small-breasted women, large-breasted women
    a. can feed at more variable intervals.
    b. can store larger volumes of milk.
    c. generally feed their infant fewer times per day.
    d. generally produce more milk per day.

23. As compared with well-nourished mothers, poorly nourished (but not starved) mothers generally produce
    a. about the same average amount of breastmilk.
    b. breastmilk deficient in protein.
    c. larger quantities of breastmilk, which make up for a lower calorie density.
    d. smaller volumes of breastmilk.

24. An infant's total intake of breastmilk during the entire course of breastfeeding is most closely (and directly) correlated with
    a. birth weight.
    b. frequency of nursing.
    c. infant weight at 1 month.
    d. maternal parity.

25. Infants typically gain about _____ ounces per week during the first 4 weeks.
    a. 4
    b. 7
    c. 10
    d. 13

26. Which of the statements below is *not* true? As compared with infants fed manufactured milks, exclusively breastfed infants
    a. have similar head circumference.
    b. on average are not quite as long.
    c. weigh distinctly less between 4 and 18 months.
    d. weigh the same or somewhat more during the first 3 to 4 months.

27. As compared with small-for-gestational-age infants fed a standard formula designed for term infants, small-for-gestational-age infants who are fully breastfed
    a. are at higher risk for failure to thrive.
    b. are slightly stunted at 12 months of age.
    c. grow faster (more "catch-up" growth).
    d. typically become anemic.

28. An unaccustomed pale red tinge to breastmilk is *least* likely to have its source in
    a. an underlying maternal medical problem such as high blood pressure.
    b. bleeding in the milk ducts.
    c. red foods ingested by the mother.
    d. red medications ingested by the mother.

29. Breastmilk composition among all women varies
    a. considerably between women in farming cultures and women in industrial cultures.
    b. considerably if diet changes seasonally.
    c. little as long as calorie intake exceeds about 1,200 calories per day.
    d. little whether they are well nourished or poorly nourished.

30. The fat concentration in breastmilk is
    a. different at different times in the course of lactation.
    b. inversely related to the frequency of breastfeeding.
    c. more or less uniform throughout the course of lactation.
    d. stable both within a given mother and between mothers of similar nutritional status.

31. The variety of fatty acids in breastmilk is
    a. not affected by maternal diet.
    b. the most variable component in breastmilk.
    c. the same as in manufactured infant milks—largely long-chain polyunsaturated fatty acids.
    d. unrelated to the mild odor of breastmilk stools.

32. The concentration of cholesterol is higher in breastmilk than formula, and it is _____ in the serum of _____
    a. about the same / young formula-fed infants and in young breastfed infants.
    b. higher / adults who were breastfed.
    c. lower / adults who were breastfed.
    d. lower in / young breastfed infants than in formula-fed infants.

33. To increase the amount of fat (and thus calories) ingested by an infant at a given feeding, a mother should
    a. delay feedings until her breasts feel quite full.
    b. encourage frequent feedings regardless of how empty or full her breasts feel.
    c. let the baby finish the first breast first.
    d. switch between breasts two or three times.
    e. Only b and c.
    f. Only b and d.

34. The carbohydrate content of breastmilk is
    a. highly variable in concentration.
    b. increases from beginning to end of a feeding.
    c. indigestible until converted by lactase.
    d. largely galactose.

35. Lactose intolerance typically
    a. develops progressively after weaning.
    b. is caused by lactase in the intestinal mucosa.
    c. is most prevalent in adults of northern European descent.
    d. refers to some babies' inability to synthesize lactose.

36. The protein content of breastmilk is used
    a. for infant growth.
    b. for infant activity.
    c. to support the infant's immune response.
    d. Only a and c.
    e. Only a, b, c.

37. Of the principal proteins (whey and casein) in human milk, the concentration of whey is
    a. higher than casein in early lactation, and provides an easily digested nutrient source.
    b. higher than casein in later lactation and fuels the greater activity of the older infant.
    c. lower than casein in the breastmilk of mothers of premature infants.
    d. nearly the same as casein throughout lactation.

38. As compared with mature breastmilk, colostrum contains a _____ concentration of _____.
    a. higher / essential amino acids.
    b. higher / lactose.
    c. lower / IgA and lactoferrin.
    d. lower / protein.

39. During the course of lactation, the concentration of fat-soluble vitamins in human milk generally
    a. decreases.
    b. increases.
    c. becomes less dependent on maternal diet.
    d. becomes more strongly dependent on maternal diet.

40. Fully breastfed infants receive sufficient amounts of the following vitamins with the possible *exception* of
    a. K.
    b. E.
    c. D.
    d. A.

41. Which statement below is *not* true? Vitamin B_{12} is
    a. fat soluble and thus dependent on maternal diet.
    b. known to foster early development of an infant's central nervous system.
    c. likely to be deficient in breastmilk of mothers who do not eat meat or dairy foods.
    d. water soluble and thus dependent on maternal diet.

42. Which of the following situations produce higher than usual sodium concentrations in breastmilk?
    a. Allergic reactions in the mother such as hay fever
    b. Mastitis or abrupt weaning
    c. Onset of lactogenesis II
    d. Sudden high frequency of nursings ("growth spurts")

43. During their first 9 months or so, fully breastfed infants generally maintain an adequate iron status
    a. because breastmilk contains a relatively high (> 3.5 mg/l) concentration of iron.
    b. by utilizing iron stored in body tissue during gestation.
    c. if supplemented with iron in the same amounts supplied to formula-fed infants.
    d. with the aid of lactase, which facilitates absorption, in human milk.

44. Adding iron to an otherwise fully breastfed infant's diet
    a. is unnecessary because breastmilk contains a high concentration of iron.
    b. helps bones calcify more strongly.
    c. impairs the effectiveness of the anti-infective agent lactoferrin.
    d. improves the baby's ability to stay well oxygenated.

45. Breastfed infants are less likely than formula-fed infants to be deficient in calcium because the calcium concentration in breastmilk is
    a. about the same as formula, but breastfed infants absorb calcium better.
    b. higher than in bovine milk.
    c. low, but infants absorb it at a much higher rate than do formula-fed infants.
    d. low, but young infants also rely on calcium stores laid down in utero.

46. As compared with milk of a mother of a full-term infant, the mother of a premature infant has milk that has a _____ concentration of _____.
    a. higher / protein.
    b. higher / vitamins.
    c. lower / anti-inflammatory agents.
    d. lower / calories.

47. Breastmilk has been called "white blood" because it
    a. carries oxygen that helps keep the baby well oxygenated.
    b. contains anti-infective properties similar to those in blood.
    c. seeps or flows from an orifice in the skin.
    d. thickens and forms a "skin" when left to dry.

48. Water makes up about what percentage of human milk?
    a. 67
    b. 73
    c. 81
    d. 88

49. Staphylococci and streptococci have been isolated from breastmilk of healthy mothers. All of the following statements are true *except*
    a. any bacteria present are considered potentially harmful to the infant.
    b. the small quantities of these bacteria in breastmilk stimulate the infant's immune system.
    c. these bacteria pose less risk to the infant if they are derived from colonization by the mother's skin.
    d. they are especially active in a useful way in the gastrointestinal tract.

50. Which of the following statements is *false*? Breastmilk reduces the likelihood and severity of diarrhea
    a. by minimizing consumption of other foods that may be contaminated.
    b. by providing anti-infective agents such as lactoferrin and lysozyme.
    c. in less developed nations and also in industrialized nations.
    d. until formula or table foods are added to the diet.

51. Strong evidence shows that the protective effects of breastfeeding extend to all of the following *except*
    a. ear infection.
    b. food allergies.
    c. respiratory infections other than respiratory syncytial virus (RSV).
    d. respiratory syncytial virus (RSV).

52. An exclusively breastfed infant is less apt to have an allergic reaction, then or later, because allergenic molecules are
    a. enveloped in milk fats and rendered harmless.
    b. sequestered in the infant's liver.
    c. unable to pass through the intestinal wall.
    d. unfolded by breastmilk in the stomach.

53. The most potent allergen that a young infant is apt to encounter is
    a. heat-treated cow milk proteins (as in formula).
    b. medium-chain fats in cow milk (not heat treated).
    c. pollen in honey.
    d. proteins in cow milk (not heat treated).

54. Breastmilk influences the infant's immune system by
    a. conferring passive immunity that persists into early childhood.
    b. erasing the immune system's long-term memory.
    c. increasing the infant's white blood cell count as long as he continues to breastfeed.
    d. stimulating an active immune response.

55. White blood cells in human milk
    a. are ineffective against viruses, which live within other cells.
    b. increase in concentration until about 4 months postpartum.
    c. principally comprise phagocytes and lymphocytes.
    d. serve principally as a substrate for synthesis of other proteins.

56. Secretory IgA is
    a. ingested in markedly smaller dosages from breastmilk than from colostrum.
    b. manufactured by the placenta and stored in the maternal breast.
    c. present in lower concentration in mothers whose infants have chronic infections.
    d. the most widely active immunoglobulin in human secretions.

57. A breastfed infant who has a systemic infection is apt to have a mother whose breastmilk contains _____ than usual concentrations of _____.
    a. higher / IgA.
    b. higher / bacteria.
    c. lower / lymphocytes.
    d. lower / protein.

58. IgA in breastmilk
    a. eliminates microbes such as staphylococci that might harm the infant.
    b. is almost entirely absorbed into the infant's system through the small intestine.
    c. is commonly found in abundance in newborn feces.
    d. stimulates an active immune response in the recipient infant.

59. The intestinal environment of a fully breastfed infant discourages the proliferation of coliform bacteria because
    a. coliform bacteria are sequestered by adhesion to the intestinal wall.
    b. gram-positive lactobacilli are only minor fecal flora.
    c. growth of a lactobacilli-promoting factor is inhibited.
    d. the intestinal pH is low.

60. Lysozyme in breastmilk
    a. helps to protect the infant from inhaled allergens.
    b. increases in concentration beginning about 6 months postpartum.
    c. is present in about the same concentration as in cow milk.
    d. modifies digestive action in the stomach such that gastroesophageal reflux is minimized.

61. Infant digestion is promoted by amylase, an enzyme that breaks down starches and
    a. begins to be synthesized by the infant at about 6 months.
    b. is present in breastmilk and in cow milk.
    c. is stored in the newborn but not released until about 6 months of age.
    d. to a lesser degree, fats.

62. Mothers whose family has a history of allergies should be encouraged to do all of the following *except*
    a. avoid any cow-milk formula supplements.
    b. breastfeed for at least a year to maintain the infant's nutritional status.
    c. eliminate any food from her diet that seems to be associated with an upset baby.
    d. offer solid foods as early as 4 months but in minute quantities, to desensitize the infant.

63. In terms of typical daily rate of synthesis and volume of milk produced, a given mother's breasts
    a. are more or less the same.
    b. differ in both rate of synthesis and volume produced.
    c. each produces about the same volume but at different rates of synthesis.
    d. produces more milk from the left breast, where the baby is more commonly held.

Discussion Questions

1. Why is human milk sometimes referred to as "white blood"?

2. How does each of the following factors affect breastmilk composition and volume?
   - Gestational age of the infant
   - Mother's age
   - Beginning of the feed
   - End of the feed
   - Age of the infant

3. It has been reported that breastfed infants, as compared with infants fed manufactured milks, consume approximately 30,000 fewer kcal by 8 months of age. Of what significance to the individual baby is this finding? Of what significance is this finding to overall infant health?

4. During an exclusively breastfed infant's first four months of life, the number of kilocalories he ingests per kilogram of weight decreases markedly. Does this observation relate principally to maternal capacity for producing milk? Does this observation relate principally to infant metabolism or infant growth rate?

5. Briefly discuss the role of human milk in reducing infant morbidity and mortality resulting from
   - Diarrhea
   - Gastrointestinal infection
   - Upper respiratory infection

6. What is the bifidus factor? How does it protect the breastfeeding infant's gut?

7. What is the relationship between lactoferrin and iron? What is the mechanism by which exogenous iron may reduce lactoferrin's capacity to function?

8. By what mechanisms does breastmilk reduce the likelihood of an allergic reaction in an infant? Explain at least four mechanisms.

9. What is the primary nutritional role of each of the following compounds? How do suboptimal amounts of each affect infant health?
   - Fat-soluble vitamins
   - Iron
   - Protein
   - Water-soluble vitamins
   - Zinc

10. What is the relation between the concentration of immunoglobulins in colostrum and in mature breastmilk? From which secretion does the infant obtain the greatest volume of immunoglobulins?

11. Taurine has been added to some manufactured baby milks. Is the effectiveness of taurine in manufactured milks the same as in breastmilk? Why or why not?

12. Given 15 minutes to talk, what three main points would you make about human milk to grandmothers who will help care for a breastfeeding grandchild? Medical students who need to know all the biochemistry as well as clinically important information? Physician assistant students who need clinically important information? Women who are pregnant with a first child?

Drug Therapy and Breastfeeding

Introduction

Mother is ill; baby is breastfeeding. Where is the balance point between treating the mother and perhaps forgoing breastfeeding, or maintaining breastfeeding and perhaps risking the mother's health? A firm grounding in the pharmacokinetics of drug uptake into milk, the concentration of drug that reaches the infant, and how an infant metabolizes the drug will help the lactation consultant judge the risks involved. Questions in this chapter will help you to assess your understanding of this body of knowledge and how it applies to professional practice.

IBLCE Disciplines

Information in this chapter applies to the following disciplines tested on the certification examination offered by the International Board of Lactation Consultant Examiners: E = Maternal and Infant Pathology; F = Maternal and Infant Pharmacology and Toxicology; 4 = Prematurity; 5 = 0–2 days; 12 = General Principles.

Multiple-Choice Questions

1. During the first two days or so after childbirth, alveolar cells in the breast are _____, and proteins pass from maternal plasma into colostrum _____.

   a. large / easily.

   b. large / only with great difficulty.

   c. small / easily.

   d. small / only with difficulty.

2. Which of the following promotes a given drug's transfer into human milk?

   a. Greater tendency to bind to proteins

   b. Lesser tendency to dissolve in fats

   c. Low concentration in maternal plasma

   d. Lower molecular weight

3. The transfer of most drugs into human milk is facilitated by

   a. active transport.

   b. an impermeable alveolar membrane.

   c. ionized or bound compounds.

   d. passive diffusion.

4. The total dosage of a protein-bound drug that is transferred from a mother to her breastfeeding infant during the first 2 days postpartum is most likely to be _____, because _____.

   a. large / junctions between alveoli are open.

   b. large / protein-bound drugs are more likely to appear in colostrum.

   c. small / diffusion is not particularly efficient.

   d. small / the volume of colostrum ingested is small.

5. Maternal drugs that have a higher concentration in milk than in plasma are

   a. evidence of an active-transport or a trapping mechanism.

   b. limited to drugs that have a pH well below 7.

   c. quite common.

   d. typically high-molecular-weight drugs.

6. Maternal medications can

   a. be cleared from breastmilk only by pumping for a time interval that is twice the half-life of the last dose.

   b. be trapped in breastmilk because the alveolar membrane is porous only in the "inbound" direction.

   c. diffuse from breastmilk to plasma as plasma concentration falls.

   d. move from breastmilk back into plasma only before tight junctions close between alveolar cells.

7. To minimize the infant dosage of a maternal medication, use a medication that has a _____ half-life and is taken immediately _____ a feeding.

   a. long / after

   b. long / before

   c. short / after

   d. short / before

8. The rate of diffusion through alveolar cell membranes is _____ for compounds with a molecular weight _____ daltons.

   a. fastest / greater than 800

   b. fastest / less than 300

   c. slowest / of 300 to 800

   d. slowest / less than 300

9. Compounds whose molecular weight exceeds _____ daltons are unlikely to pass into breastmilk.

   a. 300

   b. 500

   c. 800

   d. 1,000

10. A maternal medication with which of the following characteristics will pass most readily into breast-milk?

    a. High lipid solubility, low molecular weight

    b. Low lipid solubility, low molecular weight

    c. Not protein bound, high molecular weight

    d. Protein bound, moderately lipid soluble

11. A drug described as having a high milk/plasma ratio is usually _____ for a fully breastfed infant *if* _____.

    a. safe / the infant is older than 6 months.

    b. safe / the maternal plasma concentration is low.

    c. unsafe / it has a short half-life.

    d. unsafe / the infant is less than 6 weeks old.

12. The factor *least* likely to affect drug concentration in maternal plasma is the

    a. degree of protein binding by the drug.

    b. dose administered.

    c. half-life of the drug.

    d. lipid solubility of the drug.

13. As concentration of a drug peaks in maternal plasma, the drug's concentration in breastmilk typically is

    a. high, if the drug is not well absorbed by the mother.

    b. low, because most of the drug is in maternal plasma.

    c. low, if the drug has a very long half-life.

    d. near its peak, because diffusion correlates the two.

14. Some medications are poorly absorbed into a mother's circulation for all of the following reasons *except* that the medication is

    a. applied topically.

    b. bound by IgG in the small intestine.

    c. degraded in the stomach.

    d. metabolized by the liver.

15. To estimate the dosage of a drug transferred to an infant through breastmilk, the *most* important factors to know are the drug's

    a. actual concentration in breastmilk and volume of breastmilk ingested.

    b. maximum concentration in breastmilk and infant bioavailability.

    c. milk/plasma ratio and half-life.

    d. molecular weight and maternal dosage.

16. The greatest dosage of maternal medication is transferred to a
    a. 3-month-old infant who is taking close to 1 liter per day of mother's milk.
    b. 1-month-old baby who is nursing 10 times in 24 hours.
    c. 4-day-old neonate who is breastfeeding well but not yet stooling very often.
    d. 36-week-old fetus linked by the placenta to her mother.

17. Lipid-soluble drugs may be a good choice for a breastfeeding mother of a newborn because those drugs
    a. produce a low milk/plasma ratio.
    b. tend to be excreted in infant feces.
    c. typically have short half-lives.
    d. usually are applied topically.

18. As compared with full-term neonates, preterm infants
    a. bind or metabolize drugs more quickly, which lessens their therapeutic effect.
    b. clear medications from the body more slowly.
    c. require higher dosages to achieve the same therapeutic effect.
    d. respond similarly to medications.

19. The safety of a maternal drug for a breastfeeding infant depends on all of the following *except* the drug's
    a. ease of clearance by the infant.
    b. inherent toxicity.
    c. likelihood of being bound by maternal dietary fats.
    d. maternal and infant bioavailability.

20. Caffeine in breastmilk may result in a jittery neonate because it
    a. clears only slowly in the neonate.
    b. has a high milk/plasma ratio.
    c. passes into breastmilk in high concentration.
    d. typically has low oral bioavailability.

21. A breastfeeding infant is apt to receive a larger dosage of a maternal drug if the drug is
    a. applied topically.
    b. given as a single dose.
    c. given as several sequenced doses.
    d. present in low concentration in maternal plasma.

22. The fully breastfed infant likely to receive the largest dosage of a maternal drug in breastmilk is
    a. 12 months old, because table foods in his diet may make the intestinal mucosa more permeable.
    b. 6 months old, because milk volume consumed is near its maximum.
    c. 3 to 8 days old, because abundant milk is available.
    d. Less than 2 days old, because alveolar junctions are still open.

23. To minimize the amount of maternal drug ingested by a breastfeeding infant, a mother should *avoid*

    a. expressing milk during the course of medication and saving it for later use.

    b. feeding milk stored before she began taking medication.

    c. ingesting medications with high molecular weight or high protein-binding capacity.

    d. taking a medication considered safe for infants.

24. Breastmilk secretion may be inhibited by all of the following *except*

    a. bromocriptine.

    b. estrogen.

    c. fenugreek.

    d. progestogen.

25. Contraceptives that contain estrogen or progestogen

    a. are best begun in the immediate postpartum to help ameliorate hormonal mood swings.

    b. are more likely to reduce breastmilk volume if begun in the early postpartum.

    c. may reduce breastmilk fat content even if delayed for several weeks postpartum.

    d. may increase breastmilk volume if delayed until at least 4 months postpartum.

26. To increase the milk supply of mothers of premature infants, a dopamine antagonist such as meto-clopramide

    a. acts by inhibiting dopamine release from the anterior pituitary.

    b. can be helpful in mothers who have a low plasma prolactin concentration.

    c. can be helpful in mothers who have a moderate plasma prolactin concentration.

    d. promotes the secretion of prolactin in the posterior pituitary.

27. An infant born to a mother who received methadone during her pregnancy is apt to

    a. be born after a rapid labor.

    b. delay stooling for several days.

    c. exhibit withdrawal symptoms as a newborn.

    d. have low-set ears.

28. Penicillins and cephalosporins have been measured in breastmilk in concentrations that

    a. are about 5 percent of the mother's dosage.

    b. are more than 10 percent of the mother's dosage.

    c. are trace concentration only.

    d. vary inversely with the number of days that the mother has taken the medication.

29. Clinical postpartum depression is best treated by

    a. an antidepressant with minimal side effects, because a depressed mother may not adequately care for her infant.

    b. a medication that will increase prolactin concentration to take advantage of its calming influence.

    c. general support, because nearly all psychotropic drugs put breastfeeding at risk.

    d. general support, because the side effects of psychotropic drugs in the mother would make adequate mothering difficult.

30. In a breastfeeding mother, a thyroid supplement such as thyroxine
    a. appears in moderately high concentration in breastmilk.
    b. is not contraindicated for a short course of breastfeeding (about 6 weeks) but is contraindicated for a longer term.
    c. typically produces normal plasma thyroxine concentration, and thus is safe for the baby.
    d. will make her infant more wakeful and fussy.

31. Most drugs of abuse pass readily into all of the following *except* the
    a. infant brain, risking infant sedation, apnea, or death.
    b. infant oral mucosa, causing persistent ulcers.
    c. maternal and infant plasma.
    d. maternal breastmilk.

32. All of the following statements about maternal use of radiolabeled compounds are true *except* that maternal use
    a. is always contraindicated until her infant is weaned.
    b. is facilitated by the short half-life of most of those compounds.
    c. is most hazardous for iodine-131, which concentrates in breastmilk.
    d. usually requires only brief interruption of breastfeeding and discarding of pumped milk.

33. Which of the following statements is true? Most drugs
    a. are contraindicated in the breastfeeding mother.
    b. have low, subclinical concentrations in human milk.
    c. if taken by mouth, are destroyed in the mother's stomach.
    d. pass into human milk in concentrations of clinical concern.

Discussion Questions

1. What characteristics regulate the passage of drug molecules into breastmilk?
2. Describe at least three reliable sources of information about drug use during lactation.
3. What are at least four strategies for reducing a breastfeeding infant's exposure to a medication ingested by his mother?
4. Would you be concerned about the effects on her 2-day-old infant of a sleep medication used by a new mother? Why or why not? Would your degree of concern for the infant be the same if the mother used the same medication 2 months later? Why or why not?
5. A breastfeeding mother with a 2-week-old baby asks you if she should continue to take pain pills intended to relieve the pain following a cesarean section. What do you tell this mother? What is your rationale?
6. A mother presents with nipples that are red and extremely painful. She has been taking an antibiotic for a month since her cesarean section. What do you suspect to be the culprit? Why? What do you recommend?
7. A mother of a 6-week-old breastfeeding infant asks you if she can use a bronchodilator containing ephedrine to control asthma. What do you tell the mother? What is your rationale?
8. Do topical agents, such as those used to reduce the discomfort of poison ivy, appear in breastmilk in clinically relevant amounts? If the nursing baby has begun solids already, is it better to use the topical agent and wean the baby? Why or why not?

Viruses and Breastfeeding

Introduction

Because human milk is a highly cellular fluid, it transmits viruses (which replicate inside cells); however, it also transmits antibodies that help the infant resist those viruses. A lactation consultant must understand the natural history of transmission of viruses from mother to child and how the modes of transmission and effect on the infant differ in the pregnant and the breastfeeding mother. Questions in this chapter will help you to assess your understanding of this body of information and how it applies to professional practice.

IBLCE Disciplines

Information in this chapter applies to the following disciplines tested on the certification examination offered by the International Board of Lactation Consultant Examiners: E = Maternal and Infant Pathology; F = Maternal and Infant Pharmacology and Toxicology; K = Breastfeeding Equipment; 4 = Prematurity; 5 = 0–2 days; 12 = General Principles.

Multiple-Choice Questions

1. The transmission of viral infections through breastmilk is facilitated by its high content of
    a. cells, inside of which viruses replicate.
    b. long-chain fatty acids, which provide viruses with their preferred energy substrate.
    c. protein, to which viruses bind.
    d. water, which allow viruses to move into the general circulation.

2. The transmission of cytomegalovirus through breastmilk is apt to be harmless to an infant, if maternal infection occurs

   a. after childbirth but before the mother's milk comes in, because the volume of colostrum ingested by the infant is small.

   b. during pregnancy, because the virus induces the mother to produce antibodies.

   c. long before the pregnancy, because during pregnancy maternal antibodies circulate in the absence of the virus.

   d. 3 weeks or more after delivery, because the baby's immune system is capable by that time.

3. In the United States, transmission of human immunodeficiency virus (HIV) has declined since 1991 because of all of the following interventions *except*

   a. avoidance of breastfeeding.

   b. isolation of the infant from the mother for 72 hours after delivery.

   c. routine screening of pregnant women for HIV.

   d. use of antiretroviral drugs to combat HIV.

4. The transmission of HIV through breastmilk is hindered by _____, because the _____.

   a. early feedings of both breastmilk and formula / concentration of ingested virus is thus reduced.

   b. early feedings of both breastmilk and solids / solids promote the maturation of the infant's immune system.

   c. exclusive breastfeeding / infant's intestinal mucosa is more apt to remain intact.

   d. exclusive breastfeeding / iron in the infant's gastrointestinal tract binds and inactivates viruses.

5. In developing nations, the exclusively breastfed infant of an HIV-positive mother is more likely to remain HIV-free *primarily* because factors in breastmilk

   a. bind HIV-containing cells so that they can be excreted.

   b. cause the intestinal mucosa to remain intact.

   c. confer immunologic protection to the infant.

   d. include vitamin A.

6. Which of the following is *not* a practice recommended by the U.S. Department of Health and Human Services or the World Health Organization for HIV-positive mothers?

   a. Exclusive formula feeding where it is safe and affordable

   b. Exclusive breastfeeding where replacement feeding is neither safe nor affordable

   c. Partial breastfeeding after solids are introduced

   d. Total replacement feeding (formula or formula and solids) after exclusive breastfeeding ends

7. Which of the following factors need *not* be evaluated when one assesses the risk that a breastfed baby is now positive for HIV?

   a. Duration during which the baby has breastfed

   b. Infant birth percentile for length as compared with current percentile for length

   c. Lesions in baby's mouth or on mother's nipple

   d. Timing of maternal primary infection

8. Universal precautions, designed to protect healthcare workers from infection through contact with patients, apply to
   a. blood, human milk, and semen.
   b. human milk, semen, and vaginal secretions.
   c. semen, vaginal secretions, and blood.
   d. vaginal secretions, human milk, and blood.

9. To ensure the safety of the infant carried by a woman who is positive for herpes simplex virus, vaginal delivery is *contraindicated* if
   a. herpes virus was acquired early during this pregnancy.
   b. maternal genital herpes blisters are present at delivery.
   c. mother has been positive for herpes for several years.
   d. no "ifs"—under all circumstances.

10. Mother-to-child transmission of herpes simplex virus-1 after delivery is *most likely* to be associated with
    a. even a small concentration of virus in the milk.
    b. infant contact with lesions on the mother's breast.
    c. inhalation of maternal respiratory droplets that contain herpes virus.
    d. poor handwashing by the mother after the mother stools.

11. A herpes simplex virus infection is most likely to harm the infant if the mother was first infected when the infant
    a. is a newborn.
    b. is about 6 months old and taking maximal amounts of milk.
    c. has recently weaned completely from the breast.
    d. is of any age; age has nothing to do with the seriousness of the illness.

12. After the initial manifestation of herpes virus infection, which typically is severe and painful, the virus retreats into host cells and
    a. continues promoting formation of herpes blisters nearly continuously.
    b. flares up in attenuated form at various intervals for about 15 years.
    c. flares up in attenuated form at various intervals for the rest of the person's life.
    d. gradually loses its ability to maintain itself as the host-cell defenses gain strength.

13. The breastfeeding mother of a young infant should do what after she receives a diagnosis of rubella?
    a. Continue breastfeeding.
    b. Continue breastfeeding, but discontinue if the infant tests positive for rubella.
    c. Discontinue breastfeeding to avoid the contact with lesions that might bring on rubella symptoms in her infant.
    d. Discontinue breastfeeding because rubella virus is passed through breastmilk to a breastfeeding infant.

14. A mother should be allowed to feed her newborn if she has
    a. hepatitis B but not if she has hepatitis C.
    b. hepatitis C but not if she has hepatitis B.
    c. either hepatitis B or hepatitis C.
    d. hepatitis B or hepatitis C but only if infection is acquired shortly after delivery.

15. Infants born to women infected with hepatitis B virus should
    a. breastfeed, because breastfeeding lowers the mother's plasma concentration of this virus.
    b. breastfeed, because infants not breastfed are more likely to contract the disease.
    c. *not* breastfeed, because breastfed infants of infected mothers have a higher rate of hepatitis B infection.
    d. *not* breastfeed, because the virus will compromise the infant's immature liver.

16. Which of the following viruses is almost always considered to contraindicate breastfeeding?
    a. Hepatitis C
    b. Herpes simplex
    c. HTLV-1
    d. Rubella

17. Breastfed infants receive passive immunity in utero and through breastmilk to many childhood diseases. That immunity persists
    a. for about 3 to 6 weeks.
    b. for about 3 to 6 months.
    c. during the period of exclusive breastfeeding.
    d. during the period of any breastfeeding.

Discussion Questions

1. Where do viruses replicate? How does this site influence the modes of transmission of viral illnesses?

2. Under what circumstances might a mother with herpes zoster continue to breastfeed her infant?

3. How is it that rubella can cause birth defects but is of no concern if it appears in breastmilk?

4. Does breastfeeding appear to increase the risk of hepatitis B infection in infants? What is the rationale for your answer?

5. Should a mother with a known viral infection (other than HIV) breastfeed her newborn? What is the rationale for your response?

6. What is passive immunity?

7. What are current recommendations about whether a mother with HIV should breastfeed? What considerations govern those recommendations?

8. How does the relative timing of a woman's initial HIV infection and the index pregnancy (the pregnancy being evaluated now) affect the risk of transmission to the infant? When is the risk of transmission highest? When is risk of transmission lowest?

9. Create a table like the one below, and evaluate the ways in which the listed viruses are similar and the ways in which they differ.

Virus	Route of Transmission	Likelihood of Intrapartum or Neonatal Infection	Acute or Chronic Infection	Prevention of Cross-Contamination Between Mother and Infant
Chickenpox				
Cytomegalovirus				
Hepatitis B				
Hepatitis C				
Herpes simplex				
Herpes zoster				
HIV				
HTLV-1				
Rubella				

10. On the basis of the chart created in Question 9, draw some conclusions about the advisability of breastfeeding by a mother who has a viral infection. Does the age of the infant make a difference? Explain.

11. Compare hepatitis B and hepatitis C with regard to:
    - Likelihood of transmission to the fetus
    - Likelihood of transmission through breastfeeding
    - Whether breastfeeding should be initiated or (depending on the circumstances) continued
    - Potential for protection of the child later in life
    - Potential for later chronic illnesses as a result of exposure to the virus as a fetus or newborn

12. Should a mother with an episode of active herpes at the time she delivers breastfeed her newborn? Should she room-in with her infant? Why or why not?

13. What precautions should a lactation consultant take when she assists an HIV-positive mother who is experiencing breast engorgement?

14. Should a mother who contracts chickenpox while breastfeeding wean her infant? What is the rationale for your answer?

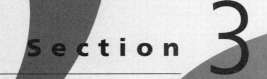

Section 3

Prenatal, Perinatal, and Postnatal Periods

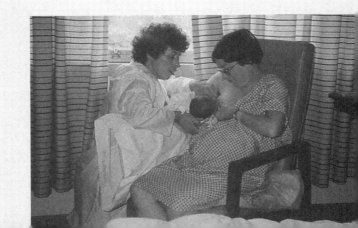

Perinatal and Intrapartum Care

Introduction

Breastfeeding cannot continue unless it is successfully begun. Thus, how to help a mother and her new baby initiate breastfeeding, whether in normal or in difficult circumstances, is of primary importance. Questions in this chapter will help you to assess your understanding of this body of information and how it applies to professional practice.

IBLCE Disciplines

Information in this chapter applies to the following disciplines tested on the certification examination offered by the International Board of Lactation Consultant Examiners: E = Maternal and Infant Pathology; H = Growth Parameters and Developmental Milestones; K = Breastfeeding Equipment and Technology; L = Techniques; 2 = Prenatal; 3 = Perinatal; 4 = Prematurity; 5 = 0–2 days; 6 = 3–14 days.

Multiple-Choice Questions

1. As compared with women who labor alone, a woman in labor who is continuously attended by a birth coach (doula) is characterized by all of the following *except* that she

    a. establishes breastfeeding sooner.

    b. is less likely to have a cesarean delivery.

    c. needs greater amounts of analgesics.

    d. labors a shorter time before baby is born.

2. A baby's mouth must shape his mother's nipple into a teat in preparation for breastfeeding. Therefore, prenatal preparation of nipples is

    a. essential only for women whose nipples are inverted.

    b. recommended for all mothers.

    c. unnecessary because colostrum taken in the early postpartum makes the nipples more elastic.

    d. not necessary because nipples become more elastic during pregnancy.

3. Benefits to the infant of breastfeeding in the first hour after birth include all of the following *except*

    a. colonization of the newborn's nose and throat with mother's benign skin bacteria.

    b. helping the infant develop his sucking reflex.

    c. prompt exposure to the immunological benefits of colostrum.

    d. reduction in the likelihood of jaundice by promoting elimination of meconium.

4. Benefits to the mother of early and frequent breastfeeding in the neonatal period include all of the following *except*

    a. acceleration of onset of lactogenesis II.

    b. reduction in breast engorgement.

    c. reduction in maternal blood loss after delivery.

    d. reduction in the rate of milk synthesis.

5. Breastfeeding helps the baby adapt to extrauterine life by all of the following *except*

    a. diminishing crying.

    b. diminishing gastric pH.

    c. increasing blood glucose.

    d. increasing skin temperature.

6. Frequent breastfeeding in the early postpartum

    a. allows milk synthesis to proceed slowly.

    b. maintains residual milk volume in the breast at a high level.

    c. promotes attachment between mother and infant.

    d. Only b and c.

7. Which of the following procedures, common during labor or immediately after delivery, typically delay the initiation of breastfeeding?

    a. Cesarean birth

    b. Epidural analgesia

    c. Suctioning the infant's mouth

    d. All of the above.

    e. Only a and b.

8. For the first 2 hours or so after her infant is born, a mother's *best* action is to

    a. allow family who attended the birth the joy of holding the baby, who will be in a quiet alert state.

    b. hold the baby skin to skin and let him nuzzle or root at the breast at will.

    c. rest as much as possible while the baby is also sleepy.

    d. try to place her nipple and areola in the baby's mouth to imprint him on the object of suckling.

9. An infant spends most of the first 24 hours after birth in which state(s)?

    a. Awake, alert

    b. Deep sleep

    c. Light sleep

    d. Light and deep sleep

10. Frequent short feedings ("cluster feeds") in the neonatal period are *best* interpreted as a sign of

    a. feeding behavior appropriate for the infant's age.

    b. lack of milk-producing capacity in the mother.

    c. mild neurological deficit that impairs the infant's ability to focus.

    d. some medical problem in the infant that prevents him from ingesting larger volumes.

11. While the baby is learning to latch onto the breast, the *best* moment to bring him to the breast is when his

    a. eyes are closed, signaling concentration.

    b. feet are pressed against the mother's opposite arm, for increased stability.

    c. mouth is wide open, but baby is not crying.

    d. neck, shoulder, and torso are aligned.

12. When latched onto the breast, a baby's lips should be

    a. flanged outward with mucous membrane against breast skin, to achieve a seal.

    b. near the nipple shaft, to make withdrawal of milk easier.

    c. pursed, to hold the breast tightly.

    d. rolled in, to reduce the likelihood that his gums will abrade breast tissue.

13. A young infant is *best* put to breast for a feeding when he is

    a. in full cry, because then his mouth is wide open and can take a big mouthful of breast.

    b. only partly awake, because then he will not object to being handled and will take the nipple more easily.

    c. restless and fussy, because he is awake enough to feed but not apt to bite the breast.

    d. wiggling or putting fingers to mouth, because he is awake and showing signs of readiness to feed.

14. During early breastfeedings, the mother should feed a neonate

    a. for no more than 10 minutes per breast, to help avoid sore nipples.

    b. no more than every 3 hours, to prevent distending the newborn's tiny stomach.

    c. on one or both breasts, to promote the baby's self-regulation of intake.

    d. only on one breast, to ensure that the baby gets both foremilk and hindmilk.

15. Skin-to-skin care of an infant in the early postpartum leads to all of the following *except*

    a. less infant crying during needle sticks.

    b. longer duration of breastfeeding.

    c. more stable infant temperature.

    d. mother gets "touched out" and has less desire to hold her infant.

16. Of the many ways to position a baby for a breastfeeding, clinical research has shown that
    a. mothers who are carefully instructed breastfeed no longer than mothers who received no instruction.
    b. only the method that emphasizes alignment of the infant head and torso is widely effective.
    c. some methods are distinctly better than others.
    d. the best position for a given mother-infant dyad depends chiefly on the degree of recession of the infant's chin.

17. When a newborn will not latch onto the breast, his mother should first do all of the following *except*
    a. digitally examine the baby's mouth to see if he can generate oral suction.
    b. evaluate the infant oral space visually.
    c. hold the baby skin to skin.
    d. watch for wiggling, mouthing, and grimacing.

18. As the center of a baby's lower lip is lightly stroked, the baby usually opens his mouth widely and
    a. blocks his windpipe by bunching his tongue.
    b. extends his tongue.
    c. sneezes.
    d. turns his face away.

19. Which is the *least* acceptable method of hand-feeding a newborn who will not latch onto the breast?
    a. Feeding bottle
    b. Finger (tube) feeding
    c. Medicine cup
    d. Teaspoon

20. During his first 2 months or so, a baby's 24-hour intake of breastmilk should be about _____ ounces for every pound of weight.
    a. 1.0
    b. 1.5
    c. 2.0
    d. 2.5

21. To be able to extract milk efficiently from the breast, an infant needs all of the following *except* a(an)
    a. intact hard and soft palate.
    b. lips that can flange to seal onto the breast.
    c. prominent rugae on the roof of the mouth to hold the breast in place.
    d. tongue that can extend beyond the lower lip and curl up on the sides.

22. Which item below optimizes the ability of a late-preterm infant (34–36 weeks gestation) to feed well?
    a. Feeding at short intervals
    b. Gently stimulating the baby
    c. Keeping the baby slightly cool to foster alertness
    d. Skin-to-skin holding

23. If a late-preterm infant does not feed well at the breast, all of the following should happen *except*

    a. begin pumping the mother's breasts.

    b. hand-feed the mother's pumped milk to the baby.

    c. limit holding of the baby to reduce stress on his system.

    d. support the mother while the baby matures.

24. As compared with low-birth-weight infants fed by feeding bottle, cup-fed low-birth-weight infants

    a. choked and spit more.

    b. ingested less milk per feeding.

    c. maintained equivalent physiologic stability.

    d. required more time per unit volume of milk ingested.

25. It is *not* appropriate to cup-feed infants who have any of the following conditions *except*

    a. irregular respiration.

    b. poor gag reflex.

    c. recently removed oral feeding tube.

    d. well-defined states.

26. A mother who is using a silicone nipple shield to help her infant latch onto her breast should also do all of the following *except*

    a. check the baby's diapers for adequate urine and stools.

    b. give water by finger-feeding.

    c. pump her breasts if they feel overly full.

    d. weigh the baby at least twice each week.

27. The plasma glucose concentration of a breastfed infant is

    a. apt to fall somewhat, immediately after birth.

    b. inversely related to frequency of feeding.

    c. lower in formula-fed infants than in breastfed infants.

    d. stable *except* for brief fluctuations when his mother's milk comes in.

28. Which of the following conditions is *least* likely to lead to hypoglycemia in a newborn infant?

    a. Infant who is small for gestational age

    b. Infant whose gestational age is more than 40 weeks

    c. Maternal diabetes

    d. Maternal hypertension

29. As compared with mothers who give birth vaginally, mothers who give birth by cesarean section tend to initiate breastfeeding at

    a. a later time, but otherwise have an uneventful breastfeeding course.

    b. a lower rate, but wean at about the same postpartum age.

    c. a small but consistently higher rate, perhaps to compensate for the operative delivery.

    d. about the same rate, but wean infants from the breast sooner.

30. When a newborn cannot breastfeed immediately, pumping his mother's breasts during the first 36 hours postpartum will
    a. hasten lactogenesis II.
    b. have no effect on milk coming in or milk transfer.
    c. increase the mother's milk supply.
    d. increase the volume of milk later ingested by the infant.
    e. Only c and d.

31. During normal postpartum engorgement,
    a. breast tissue becomes incompressible.
    b. the baby cannot latch onto the breast.
    c. the mother may run a low fever.
    d. to protect fragile breast tissue, the breast should be offered at as long intervals as the baby will tolerate.

32. The likelihood of excessive breast engorgement is *increased* in mothers who
    a. avoid use of formula supplements.
    b. ensure that the baby feeds from both breasts at each feeding.
    c. feeds about 8 to 12 times per 24 hours.
    d. initiate breastfeeding in the early postpartum.

33. In the early weeks, the *most* reliable indicator that a baby is taking sufficient milk is that the baby
    a. is contented and rarely cries.
    b. produces several wet diapers and some stool each day.
    c. swallows audibly during much of each feeding.
    d. wakes on his own for feedings.

34. Weaning by 10 days postpartum is associated with all of the following *except*
    a. extremely short intervals between breastfeedings.
    b. three or more feedings by bottle.
    c. vaginal delivery assisted by lengthy administration of Pitocin.
    d. vaginal delivery assisted by vacuum extraction.

35. Between birth and discharge, and as compared with formula-fed infants, the percentage weight loss of breastfed infants is about
    a. 15 percent less.
    b. the same.
    c. twice as much.
    d. half as much.

36. Before discharge, first-time breastfeeding mothers should be taught about all of the following *except*
    a. infant feeding cues.
    b. latching the baby onto her breast.
    c. preparing emergency bottles of infant formula.
    d. signs of sufficient milk intake.

37. A baby should be evaluated for insufficient milk intake if he produces

    a. colorless urine at any time.

    b. sticky black or green stools before lactogenesis II is established.

    c. urine that contains red dust ("brick dust") after lactogenesis II is established.

    d. yellowish stools after lactogenesis II is established.

38. A baby should be evaluated for insufficient milk intake if his mother experiences any of the following *except* she

    a. has painful engorged breasts.

    b. hears or feels no swallowing during feedings.

    c. must wake the baby for most feeds.

    d. suddenly resolves very sore nipples.

39. Maternity ward discharge packs that contain infant formula typically affect the duration of breast-feeding how?

    a. Lengthen any breastfeeding

    b. Lengthen breastfeeding combined with supplemental foods

    c. No effect on exclusive breastfeeding

    d. Shorten exclusive breastfeeding

40. Cup-feeding of infants who are unable to latch onto the breast is more likely to be successful if the infant has which of the following characteristics?

    a. Broken clavicle

    b. Difficulty breathing

    c. Neurological delay or deficit

    d. Poor gag reflex

Discussion Questions

1. Describe at least three ways that a pregnant woman can prepare herself for breastfeeding.

2. Describe at least five faulty assumptions about breastfeeding. What is a better way to explain how breastfeeding can work in each situation?

3. Describe at least three ways to hold a baby for breastfeeding. When is each position best used? What are cautions that apply to each position?

4. What is hypoglycemia? When it is most likely to occur in a neonate? How should the baby be managed? What is the rationale for this management?

5. In a healthy newborn who displays a normal suckling pattern, what do the baby's cheeks look like? Where is the baby's tongue? Is any of it visible? What do you hear during suckling bursts? How are the baby's lips placed? How firmly is the baby attached to the breast?

6. What is finger-feeding? What are indications for its use? What are cautions about its use?

7. Describe at least three practices in the early postpartum that contribute to breast engorgement in a breastfeeding mother. Describe better practices that minimize engorgement.

8. Under what circumstances might you use a thin silicone nipple shield to assist breastfeeding? What are cautions about its use?

9. Why does early, frequent breastfeeding promote optimal functioning in both mother and newborn? Discuss at least four reasons. Show how each reason supports the other reasons you discuss.

10. How is postpartum breast fullness distinguished from breast engorgement? How is each best treated?

8

Postpartum Care

Introduction

The information in this chapter expands on that in the preceding chapter and extends into the mother's "fourth trimester." Hallmarks of successful breastfeeding are a confident, comfortable mother and a thriving infant. Questions in this chapter will help you to assess your understanding of how to help mothers and babies achieve these goals.

IBLCE Disciplines

Information in this chapter applies to the following disciplines tested on the certification examination offered by the International Board of Lactation Consultant Examiners: C = Maternal and Infant Normal Nutrition and Biochemistry; E = Maternal and Infant Pathology; F = Maternal and Infant Pharmacology and Toxicology; H = Growth Parameters and Developmental Milestones; K = Breastfeeding Equipment and Technology; L = Techniques; 3 = Perinatal; 4 = Prematurity; 5 = 0–2 days; 6 = 3–14 days.

Multiple-Choice Questions

1. The principal reasons that cause mothers to abandon breastfeeding are concerns about
   a. breasts leaking and use of pacifiers.
   b. inadequate milk supply and nipple pain.
   c. nipple pain and leaking.
   d. use of pacifiers and inadequate milk supply.

2. As compared with the average volume of a single letdown during the first week postpartum, the capacity of a week-old infant's stomach is about
    a. half again as much—about an ounce.
    b. only half as much—about an ounce.
    c. the same or a bit less—about an ounce.
    d. twice as much—about an ounce.

3. By 1 month of age, fully breastfeeding babies ingest an average daily volume of about _____ ml.
    a. 600
    b. 700
    c. 800
    d. 900

4. At feedings in which the baby sets the pace, by far the largest majority of healthy, fully breastfed infants will feed from
    a. both breasts.
    b. one breast at one feed and both breasts at the next.
    c. one breast at the early morning feeding, but both breasts in the evening.
    d. one breast only.

5. Restful maternal sleep is *best* provided by
    a. breastfeeding supplemented with one bottle during the middle of the night.
    b. exclusive bottle-feeding.
    c. exclusive breastfeeding and safe bed-sharing.
    d. exclusive breastfeeding of an infant who sleeps in his own crib.

6. When a young infant cries he is
    a. improving his oxygenation.
    b. providing an early sign of hunger.
    c. reducing his internal level of stress.
    d. strongly signaling intense hunger.

7. During the first week postpartum, milk intake by the fully breastfed infant likely is adequate if all of the following signs are present *except* baby
    a. actively suckles at least about 2.5 hours each day.
    b. feeds an average of 10 or so times a day.
    c. finishes many nursing bouts by falling asleep with the nipple in his mouth.
    d. swallows audibly while feeding.

8. Gently pinched infant skin that retains the "pinched" shape indicates
    a. an infant who is not sufficiently hydrated.
    b. Asian heritage of the infant.
    c. edema, now resolved, in the neonate.
    d. fragile skin suggesting a connective-tissue disorder.

9. A feeding that has the characteristics listed below may suggest poor milk transfer, *except*

   a. breasts still feel firm.

   b. creases on opposite sides of the nipple.

   c. mother and baby are drowsy.

   d. nipples are sore.

10. Immediate and sustained skin-to-skin contact between mother and her newborn promotes all of the following *except*

    a. abundant milk production.

    b. comfort for the newborn.

    c. maternal confidence in caring for her newborn.

    d. normal lactogenesis I.

11. An infant who does not latch onto the breast well within the first 24 hours may be reacting to all of the following *except*

    a. a forceps or extraction delivery.

    b. a small cleft of the soft palate.

    c. his mother's unmedicated labor.

    d. torticollis.

12. When a baby feeds well from one breast but refuses ever to feed from the breast on the mother's other side, the mother should do all of the following *except*

    a. express milk from the refused breast.

    b. extend the time between feedings and always offer the rejected breast first.

    c. have the baby examined for a birth injury.

    d. offer the rejected breast from time to time.

13. When an infant's suckle causes nipple pain, the *best* response is to gently

    a. dribble a glucose solution onto his lips to encourage him to reposition himself.

    b. remove baby from the breast and reposition him.

    c. shift the infant's position while leaving him attached to the breast.

    d. tickle or lightly massage his throat from chin to collarbone to encourage him to take a larger mouthful of breast.

14. When breastfeeding must be supplemented with commercial formula, all of the following are discouraged *except*

    a. commercial ready-to-feed formula, because it is sterile.

    b. straight-sided bottles, which increase the need for burping.

    c. propping the bottle, which may put the infant at greater risk of ear infections.

    d. warming the formula in the microwave oven, because hot spots in the milk may result.

15. Transient nipple soreness typically is most noticeable during days

    a. 1 and 2 postpartum.

    b. 1 through 10 postpartum.

    c. 3 through 6 postpartum.

    d. 6 through 10 postpartum.

16. When it is positioned in the mouth for comfortable milk transfer, the nipple typically
    a. becomes wedge shaped as it nearly doubles its length.
    b. elongates so that nipple pores are positioned near the soft palate.
    c. flattens between the tongue and roof of the mouth but stretches very little.
    d. rests midway between gum ridge and pharynx.

17. Nipple pain in the early postpartum is related to
    a. fair hair or skin color.
    b. lack of prenatal buffing (or other preparation) of the nipples.
    c. multiparity.
    d. all of the above.
    e. none of the above.

18. Nipple pain that persists beyond one week postpartum is
    a. abnormal and should be investigated.
    b. likely to be caused by a problem in the nipples themselves.
    c. normal in first-time breastfeeding mothers.
    d. rarely avoidable in mothers of premature or "late premature" infants.

19. A useful way to reduce nipple pain in the early days of breastfeeding is to
    a. allow the baby to comfort himself with a pacifier.
    b. at any one feeding, feed from both breasts.
    c. breastfeed for short periods only.
    d. ensure that the baby's lips and gums are well back onto the areola or breast skin.

20. During suck-swallow-breathe episodes, milk flows into the baby's mouth fastest during the
    a. downward movement of the baby's jaw.
    b. pause between suck-swallow-breathe episodes.
    c. pause for breathing.
    d. upward movement of the baby's jaw.

21. A short or tight lingual frenulum typically
    a. allows the tip of the tongue to remain pointed.
    b. improves milk transfer.
    c. restricts extension of the tongue.
    d. supports the tongue so that it can extend during latch onto the breast.

22. The *best* way to attach a full-term infant to the breast is to
    a. hold the baby skin-to-skin and allow him to attach by himself.
    b. offer a nipple that is compressed horizontally.
    c. prefer a cradle or cross-cradle position.
    d. support the infant's feet so he can steady himself.

23. A painful abraded nipple in the first few days postpartum is *best* treated by
    a. breast shells to protect nipples from abrasion by clothing.
    b. correcting the position of the infant's mouth on the breast.
    c. rubbing breastmilk into the nipple.
    d. topical antibiotics to heal any infection.
    e. Only b and c.
    f. Only b, c, and d.

24. With respect to the milk-producing cells (alveoli or lactocytes), breast engorgement combined with milk stasis typically leads to
    a. a decrease in their number.
    b. an increase in their number.
    c. an increase in their size.
    d. their involution.

25. Gentle massage of the lactating breast, common in many cultures, is thought to help do all of the following *except*
    a. delay the milk-ejection reflex.
    b. increase milk volumes.
    c. move interstitial fluid out of the breasts.
    d. soften the nipple and areola of a very firm breast.

26. An infant who makes a "clicking" sound while nursing is *most* likely to be
    a. breathing through his mouth while feeding.
    b. catching his breath between bursts of suckling.
    c. sucking on his tongue.
    d. swallowing large boluses of milk.

27. Edema in the breast tissue surrounding milk ducts appears to
    a. be associated with repair of maternal episiotomy.
    b. constrict the space available for dilation of milk ducts during milk ejection.
    c. migrate into milk ducts and increase the volume of foremilk.
    d. promote the typical thirst felt by women during a breastfeeding.

28. Engorgement, painful swelling of the breast, is produced by
    a. edema only, when interstitial fluid pinches ducts closed.
    b. either lactogenesis II or edema, or both.
    c. lactogenesis II only, when milk is synthesized more rapidly than it is removed.
    d. lactogenesis II only, when spasms in the nipple do not allow milk to flow out of the breast.

29. Abundant milk production on day 6 postpartum is
    a. a marker for a milk supply that may need reducing to keep the mother comfortable.
    b. a spike in production that will settle back once the baby is on a feeding schedule.
    c. closely associated with abundant milk production at 6 weeks postpartum.
    d. residual engorgement and will diminish in the next week or so.

30. As compared with small-breasted women, large-breasted women typically have a _____ breastmilk-storage capacity, because _____.
    a. larger / ducts and alveoli are expanded during the period of engorgement.
    b. larger / the volume of milk-producing and storage structures is larger.
    c. similar / breast size doesn't make a difference.
    d. smaller / most breast volume represents subcutaneous fat.

31. Retention of milk in the breast may be caused by all of the following *except*
    a. highly twisted or braided milk ducts.
    b. ineffective infant suckle.
    c. maternal rate of milk synthesis greater than infant rate of milk removal.
    d. sleepy baby who nurses infrequently.

32. Breasts will begin to involute when
    a. components in the milk promote proliferation of lactocytes.
    b. distention of the lumen of milk aveoli disrupts lactocytes.
    c. only about 80% of milk in the breasts is consistently removed.
    d. they consistently have excess storage capacity.

33. On average, breasts synthesize milk at the rate of _____ ml per breast per hour, but a nearly empty breast typically is _____ that rate.
    a. 20 / double
    b. 30 / double
    c. 40 / half again
    d. 50 / the same as

34. To soften a breast swollen with edema, all of the following are useful *except*
    a. cold packs for 20-minute intervals.
    b. compression of the areola
    c. gentle massage to mobilize lymph.
    d. hot packs for 20-minute intervals.

35. The maternal assertion "I don't have enough milk for the baby" is *most* likely caused by a
    a. lack of interest in breastfeeding.
    b. misinterpretation of normal newborn breastfeeding behavior.
    c. need for more uninterrupted sleep.
    d. real physical problem for a large percentage of primiparous mothers.

36. Mothers of thriving fully breastfed infants typically synthesize at least _____ percent more milk than their infants usually take.
    a. 7
    b. 12
    c. 20
    d. 33

37. Delayed lactogenesis II is associated with all of the following *except*

    a. bursts of prolactin that accompany infant suckling or breast pumping.

    b. ineffective infant suckling.

    c. insulin-dependent diabetes mellitus or obesity.

    d. stressful labor and delivery, such as a cesarean birth.

38. Infant behavior at the breast that suggests milk oversupply may also be caused by a

    a. baby who nurses too vigorously.

    b. baby who poorly coordinates feeding with breathing.

    c. breastmilk flavor unfamiliar to the infant.

    d. breast compensating for poor letdown caused by sore nipples.

39. By about 6 weeks postpartum, the mother's milk supply adjusts relative to the baby so that the

    a. baby must increase the number of feeds per day to consume enough milk.

    b. breast retains enough residual milk that supplemental feeds need to begin.

    c. breast retains sufficient residual milk to allow for occasional larger feeds.

    d. fat content of the milk is higher, and the baby will thrive on fewer feeds per day.

40. Use of pacifiers may do all of the following, *except*

    a. down-regulate maternal milk supply by reducing (by one) the number of feedings per day.

    b. during sleep, reduce the incidence of sudden unexplained infant death.

    c. during the first month, delay effective breastfeeding.

    d. encourage development of an effective latch at the breast.

41. By two weeks of age, the fecal flora in fully breastfed infants is dominated by

    a. bifidobacteria and lactobacilli.

    b. coliforms and bifidobacteria.

    c. enterococci and coliforms.

    d. lactobacilli and enterococci.

42. After about day 4 postpartum, when full breastmilk feedings are established, the neonate's stools are _____ because the proportion of _____ is _____.

    a. brown and soft / casein / high.

    b. greenish and sticky / casein / low.

    c. yellow and firm / whey / low.

    d. yellow and very soft or runny / whey / high.

43. During the first 6 months or so, the whey:casein ratio in human milk

    a. decreases from about 90:10 to about 60:40.

    b. increases from about 60:40 to about 90:10.

    c. stays constant at about 80:20.

    d. stays constant at about 50:50.

44. In the first week postpartum, frequent breastfeeding is associated with all of the following *except*
    a. copious, odorous stools.
    b. earlier appearance of yellow stools.
    c. faster weight gain.
    d. reduction of breast engorgement.

45. Which of the following statements is false? The whey portion of breastmilk contains
    a. constituents that confer immunity.
    b. factors that promote growth of long bones.
    c. small quantities of minerals.
    d. the water in breastmilk.

46. A fully breastfed infant who passes only two or three stools every 2 weeks is *most* likely to be
    a. constipated.
    b. less than 6 weeks old, when breastmilk is very watery.
    c. older than 6 weeks and metabolizing essentially all breastmilk constituents.
    d. showing symptoms of a disorder of intestinal peristalsis.

47. Breastfeeding during painful procedures, such as blood draws, on the infant typically
    a. allows blood to flow faster into the needle.
    b. makes breastfeeding more stressful on the infant at other times.
    c. reduces the infant's pain.
    d. results in biting or clamping on the nipple.

48. Slightly elevated plasma bilirubin concentration (greater than 5 milligrams per deciliter) requires no intervention beyond continued adequate feeding if the baby is
    a. also taking water supplements.
    b. less than 2 weeks old.
    c. older than 3 weeks and otherwise thriving.
    d. premature or "late premature."

49. Infant crying
    a. decreases infant blood pressure.
    b. improves overall vigor.
    c. is exacerbated by the confinement of being carried.
    d. signals a need.

50. A feeding regime regulated by the clock may result in all of the following *except*
    a. attentiveness to infant cues for cluster feedings.
    b. dehydration of the infant.
    c. reduction of maternal milk supply.
    d. underfeeding of the infant.

51. A common first response to a crying baby is to offer the breast, because the
    a. act of suckling calms the baby, in part by releasing natural endorphins.
    b. baby cannot cry and feed at the same time.
    c. caloric content of breastmilk replaces the calories expended crying, thus stabilizing the infant.
    d. mother's breast, which is slightly cooler than other skin, calms an overstimulated baby.

52. The food allergen most commonly ingested in the first year is
    a. chicken.
    b. cow milk.
    c. egg.
    d. soy (in formula).

53. A breastfeeding infant in whom symptoms of colic develop in response to allergens in his mother's diet
    a. is likely to show allergic reactions to those same foods later in life.
    b. is protected against allergic reactions to those same foods.
    c. risks other exaggerated responses to food that may lead to obesity.
    d. should be started on bland table foods as early as possible.

54. The distressing infant crying considered typical of infant colic is *best* ameliorated by
    a. carrying the baby supine on a parent's forearm.
    b. increased carrying near the heart.
    c. small sips of clear water.
    d. unwrapping the infant.

55. Lactation consultants may work with mothers of twins (or higher order newborns) because
    a. environmental factors currently make release of two or more ova more likely when mothers ovulate.
    b. multiples are more likely to be born to young mothers, who have developed less milk-secreting tissue.
    c. those infants are apt to be released from the hospital before they feed well.
    d. those mothers initiate breastfeeding at about the same rate as mothers of singletons.

56. A mother who breastfeeds her multiple infants
    a. has the milk-producing capacity to provide all or nearly all the nourishment required by twins or triplets.
    b. should begin using a pharmaceutical contraceptive as soon as she completes her 6-week postpartum checkup.
    c. will produce breastmilk in adequate volumes but diminished calorie content.
    d. will have adequate volume but diminished immunological components.

57. Near-term ("late preterm") multiple infants are more susceptible to all of the following *except*
    a. blocked tear ducts.
    b. elevated plasma bilirubin concentration.
    c. hypoglycemia.
    d. less effective suckling.

58. A subsequent conception while breastfeeding is _____ if the _____.
    a. likely / baby is fully breastfeeding and less than 6 months old.
    b. likely / mother is losing more than a pound per week of weight gained during pregnancy.
    c. unlikely / baby feeds any amount from the breast.
    d. unlikely / baby is fully breastfeeding and less than 6 months old.

59. A mother who continues to breastfeed an older child during a subsequent pregnancy is apt to experience all of the following *except*
    a. an increase in energy.
    b. breast and nipple tenderness.
    c. change in taste of her milk.
    d. smaller milk supply.

60. Continuing to breastfeed a toddler during a subsequent pregnancy should be discouraged
    a. because the older infant will be at nutritional risk.
    b. even if the mother's pregnancy is in healthy and uncomplicated.
    c. if the mother has miscarried before or is carrying twins.
    d. to avoid a typically debilitating energy demand on the mother.

61. When a breastfeeding mother and her infant share a bed at night, all of the following happen *except* that the
    a. baby feeds more frequently.
    b. mother responds to infant movements more quickly.
    c. mother tends to get less restful sleep.
    d. total duration of breastfeeding is extended.

62. The risk of unexplained sudden infant death strongly correlates with all of the following *except*
    a. a diet of infant formula.
    b. lack of carrying while awake.
    c. maternal smoking.
    d. the infant sleeping on his stomach.

63. The risk of sudden infant death may increased as much as four times if the baby is
    a. at risk because of premature birth.
    b. breastfed by a mother who smokes.
    c. placed in day care.
    d. put to sleep in his own crib from birth.

64. A baby sharing a bed with adults is most likely to be smothered by
    a. a parent whose nature is to sleep quite deeply.
    b. an adult who is not the baby's parent.
    c. an adult who has recently used alcohol or illicit drugs.
    d. the parent to whom he sleeps most closely—usually his mother.
    e. Only a and d.
    f. Only b and c.

65. Mother and her young breastfeeding infant are *best* described as

   a. a pair of people uniquely fitted to fill each other's physical needs.

   b. independent beings, after birth, who come together for their mutual advantage.

   c. individuals, each benefited by some separation from each other.

   d. two parts of a single psychological and biological organism.

Discussion Questions

1. What is the normal pattern of weight change in the first 2 weeks of an infant's life? What percent weight loss is a marker for further evaluation? What is the latest day that a baby should begin regaining weight? What is the latest day by which birth weight should be regained?

2. What are cluster feedings? Are they cause for alarm? How should they best be handled?

3. How are severe postpartum hemorrhage and later breastfeeding difficulties related?

4. Contrast typical stooling patterns in an exclusively breastfed baby and a baby exclusively fed manufactured milks at the following time points:
   • Day 2
   • Day 5
   • 2 weeks
   • 1 month
   • 3 months

5. A 3-month-old baby is at the 75th percentile for height and the 50th percentile for weight. How do you respond to a mother who thinks she doesn't have enough milk for this baby? What might the baby be doing to make the mother draw this conclusion? Discuss at least five factors. What might the mother be doing or feeling to make her draw this conclusion? Discuss at least five factors.

6. How do you decide whether "sore nipples" are transient and normal or are prolonged and abnormal? What might cause each case? What would you suggest to resolve each one?

7. Why do babies sometimes refuse the breast? Give at least three reasons; consider infants at various ages. What would you suggest to return the baby to the breast?

8. What is an overactive letdown? Is it a problem? Why or why not? How can the mother cope with it?

9. What information about breastfeeding should be discussed as part of a hospital discharge plan for a postpartum woman?

10. What community services or organizations can you recommend to a new breastfeeding mother who is now at home?

Breast-Related Problems

Introduction

Atypical physical characteristics of the breast, either temporary or permanent, can render breastfeeding difficult. This chapter describes how to recognize, manage, or compensate for atypical presentations of the exterior skin and the interior tissues of the breast that impinge upon breastfeeding. Questions in this chapter will help you to assess your understanding of this body of information and how it applies to professional practice.

IBLCE Disciplines

Information in this chapter applies to the following disciplines tested on the certification examination offered by the International Board of Lactation Consultant Examiners: B = Maternal and Infant Normal Physiology and Endocrinology; D = Maternal and Infant Immunology and Infectious Disease; L = Techniques; 2 = Prenatal; 12 = General Principles.

Multiple-Choice Questions

1. Inverted nipples that can, with effort, be pulled out are likely to
   a. be associated with clothing that binds the breasts.
   b. evert more easily with each subsequent child breastfed.
   c. maintain that degree of inversion throughout pregnancy and lactation.
   d. prevent most newborns from drawing the nipple into his mouth.

2. An inverted nipple usually _____ sufficient milk transfer, _____.
   a. permits / as long as the baby's gums are well back on the areola.
   b. permits / if the baby is positioned on his back to feed.
   c. prevents / because the infant has nothing to grasp.
   d. prevents / because most milk ducts in the nipple are pinched or kinked.

3. If a mother wishes to manipulate her flat or retracted nipples to make them easier for the infant to grasp, the best time to begin is
   a. after her milk comes in.
   b. as soon as the pregnancy is confirmed.
   c. right before the newborn's first attempt to latch.
   d. beginning in the seventh month.

4. Exceptionally long maternal nipples tend to
   a. fatigue the infant, because milk ducts are very narrow.
   b. flood the infant with milk during the initial letdown, causing him to pull off the breast.
   c. may prevent large neonates from grasping the areola.
   d. trigger a gag reflex in susceptible infants.

5. Plugged ducts are most commonly associated with a
   a. baby who rarely takes most of the milk in the breast.
   b. barely adequate milk supply that leads to many feedings, thus many letdowns.
   c. local tenderness in the affected breast and a generalized fever.
   d. palpable lump in the breast and a generalized fever.

6. To promote opening of a plugged duct, a mother is advised to
   a. begin each feed on the unaffected breast.
   b. breastfeed at longer intervals to increase milk pressure behind the plug.
   c. firmly massage the tender area after each breastfeeding.
   d. position the baby so that his nose points to the tender area.

7. A mother in whom mastitis has developed typically will experience all of the following *except*
   a. generalized fever.
   b. hot, red, tender area on one breast.
   c. muscle aching and headache.
   d. slow pulse.

8. Any one mastitis infection usually is
   a. bilateral.
   b. confined to one breast.
   c. found in the portion of the breast below the nipple.
   d. identified by red streaks that radiate from the nipple.

9. The risk of a mastitis infection is greatest
   a. about the time that solids begin to be added.
   b. before the 6-week checkup.
   c. in primiparous women.
   d. when the baby weans completely.

10. A mother may be more susceptible to a breast infection if she has all of the following *except*
   a. a cracked nipple.
   b. an ample milk supply.
   c. extreme stress or fatigue.
   d. a baby who recently increased the number of feedings per day (as in response to a growth spurt).

11. To promote recovery from a breast infection a mother is *best* advised to
   a. apply moist heat to the affected region and in the nearby axilla.
   b. avoid analgesics, which lengthen the duration of the infection.
   c. avoid unnecessary activity, and rest in bed if possible.
   d. decrease fluids, to lessen the risk of breast engorgement.

12. A mother with mastitis who temporarily stops breastfeeding
   a. allows medications used by the mother to remain in the breast longer, promoting healing.
   b. allows the breasts to overfill and thus dilute the infected fluids in the breast.
   c. delays the mother's recovery, unless she pumps as much milk as the baby normally takes.
   d. protects the baby from the risk posed by infected breastmilk.

13. During a breast infection, the composition of breastmilk changes such that lactoferrin
   a. and chloride decrease, but sodium increases.
   b. and sodium increase, but chloride decreases.
   c. sodium, and chloride all decrease.
   d. sodium, and chloride all increase.

14. After recovery from mastitis, for a short time the affected breast usually produces _____ milk than before, because _____.
   a. less / initially the baby will be reluctant to feed from that breast.
   b. less / the rate of milk synthesis in that breast is diminished.
   c. more / if the mother in fact was able to stay on bedrest during the infection.
   d. more / milk stored in alveoli is now released.

15. Inflammatory breast cancer, like mastitis, may produce a locally inflamed and swollen breast. The breast cancer is characterized by all of the following *except*
   a. causes fever only rarely.
   b. commonly produces a palpable mass.
   c. does not produce a mass that can be easily felt.
   d. does not regress with antibiotic treatment.

16. A breast abscess
    a. can be traced to streptococcal bacteria in most women.
    b. if it needs to be drained surgically, will force the end of breastfeeding on that breast.
    c. is the outcome of approximately three-quarters of cases of mastitis.
    d. may require incision and drainage, after which breastfeeding can resume.

17. The risk of painful eczema developing in a nipple increases if the mother is characterized by all of the following *except*
    a. does not wear "breathable" (such as all-cotton) brassieres.
    b. exposes her breasts and nipples to the sun.
    c. has a history of eczema.
    d. recently introduced solids to her still-breastfeeding infant.

18. A mother who has herpes simplex on her nipples is *best* advised to
    a. continue nursing but use nipple shields to protect the nipple.
    b. feed freshly pumped milk to the infant.
    c. interrupt nursing temporarily; pump and discard milk until herpes lesions are gone.
    d. nurse using nipple shields when the baby is otherwise inconsolable, but formula-feed at other times.

19. Mothers and infants who have recently received antibiotic therapy are more susceptible to
    a. candidiasis.
    b. eczema.
    c. herpes simplex.
    d. nipple rash.

20. A *Candida* infection of the breastfeeding dyad may appear as
    a. painful, deep pink nipples in the mother.
    b. red, sore-looking diaper rash in the baby.
    c. white coating in the baby's mouth.
    d. vaginal *Candida* infection in the mother.
    e. All of the above.
    f. Only a, b, and d.

21. To eliminate a breastfeeding mother's recurrent yeast infection, which of the following should be treated? The woman, _____.
    a. and her sexual partner.
    b. her sexual partner, and her infant.
    c. her sexual partner, her infant, and items that regularly touch the baby's mouth or mother's breasts
    d. and the infant's anal region only.

22. The expressed breastmilk of a mother who is currently being treated for candidiasis (a yeast infection) of the nipple is best handled by

    a. bottle feeding the fresh milk to her baby.

    b. discarding the pumped milk until she has finished treatment and is free of symptoms.

    c. freezing the milk for later bottle feeding.

    d. leaving the milk at room temperature for several hours so that factors in the milk will inactivate any yeast in it.

23. Pain deep within the breast is commonly associated with all of the following *except*

    a. damage to the surface of the nipple.

    b. forceful milk ejection and refilling of milk ducts.

    c. noninflammatory cancerous tumor.

    d. pinched nipples resulting from compression of the nipple against the infant's hard palate.

24. A typically painful "milk blister," a blister that contains milk, forms

    a. at the outlet of a nipple pore that has sealed over and blocked milk behind it.

    b. in the center of a breastfeeding baby's upper lip.

    c. on the end or side of a nipple rubbed against rugae on a baby's hard palate.

    d. within the breast proximal to a milk duct; another name is galactocele.

25. A woman who has had surgery that changed her breast size generally will have the *best* chance of breastfeeding if the

    a. blood vessels to the areola complex, rather than to lactocytes, were severed.

    b. breast was augmented rather than reduced.

    c. breast was reduced rather than augmented.

    d. first intercostal nerves were not severed.

26. After breast reduction surgery, a woman has the *least* chance of producing adequate breastmilk if the

    a. free-nipple technique of breast reconstruction was used.

    b. minimal amount of glandular tissue was removed.

    c. seventh intercostal nerve was severed.

    d. sixth intercostal nerve was severed.

27. In breast reduction surgery, removal of extra subcutaneous adipose tissue _____ milk-producing structures because _____.

    a. injures / the fat cushion around nerves is removed, and signals from the nipple to the brain are less effective.

    b. injures / the milk-producing cells must be cut to remove intergrown fat.

    c. does not injure / the fat mostly lies directly below the skin and strips out cleanly.

    d. does not injure / because most fat accumulates below the nipple and away from important ducts and nerves.

28. Breast augmentation surgery will likely result in all of the following *except*
    a. increase in first-week engorgement.
    b. normal initial milk production.
    c. reduction of the breasts' long-term ability to ramp up milk production to meet infant needs.
    d. retention of full sensation to the nipple after periareolar incision.

29. Milk ducts severed during breast reduction surgery usually _____ breastfeeding, because the severed ducts tend to _____.
    a. do not hinder / reattach to intact ducts.
    b. do not hinder / reattach to each other.
    c. hinder / spill milk into breast tissue, which is more likely to develop mastitis.
    d. hinder / seal at the severed end and cause pressure atrophy of alveoli ejecting milk into those ducts.

30. A reddish or brownish tinge to breastmilk
    a. is most common in primiparous women in the early days of breastfeeding.
    b. means that the baby should be weaned to avoid ingesting blood.
    c. reflects the thinner, more porous walls in milk ducts of multiparous women.
    d. usually means that the mother ate red foods in the previous 18 hours or so.

31. If bright red fluid issues from a nipple pore, the mother should be evaluated for a(an)
    a. extremely high blood pressure.
    b. galactocele.
    c. intraductal papilloma.
    d. plugged duct.

32. Breast cancer is *less* likely in women who breastfed at least one infant and who
    a. had menstruated at least 10 years or so at the time their first infant was born.
    b. maintain high circulating estrogen concentrations.
    c. still menstruate regularly.
    d. weaned very young infants.

33. A woman should be evaluated for breast cancer if she notes any of the following *except*
    a. bouts of mastitis that appear in various locations in the breast.
    b. breast lump that maintains its size during feedings.
    c. "plugged duct" that persists beyond three days of treatment.
    d. region of breast skin that has many small dimples, like an orange skin.

34. An infant who feeds from a cancerous breast
    a. if a girl, has no greater likelihood of cancer later developing than the general population.
    b. if a boy, is more likely to develop cancer later in life.
    c. nearly always rejects that breast in favor of the noncancerous one.
    d. rarely rejects the cancerous breast.

35. Women being treated by chemotherapy for any cancer should be encouraged to _____, because commonly used chemotherapy drugs_____.

    a. breastfeed / do pass into breastmilk but are destroyed in the infant's stomach.

    b. breastfeed / have molecules too large to pass into breastmilk.

    c. not breastfeed temporarily / do pass into breastmilk and are potentially toxic to the infant.

    d. not breastfeed at all / will not eliminate all cancerous particles and thus the breastfeeding infant is exposed to those particles.

36. As compared with the breasts of a woman who is neither pregnant nor lactating, the breasts of a lactating woman may be more difficult to evaluate for breast cancer by the use of conventional mammography for all of the following reasons *except* that her breasts

    a. are denser.

    b. contain more glandular tissue.

    c. have a higher water content.

    d. move blood more slowly.

37. Mothers who gave birth to an infant after treatment for breast cancer report all of the following *except*

    a. a nipple on the treated breast that does not stretch to its former length.

    b. diminished or absent lactation in a breast treated for a centrally located tumor.

    c. little or no enlargement of the treated breast during pregnancy.

    d. no difference in milk supply between treated and untreated breast.

38. After a breastfeeding mother has had surgery on a breast, such as a biopsy, a lump removed, or an abscess drained, her *best* response is to resume breastfeeding

    a. after a delay of 3 or 4 days, to give her body a chance to begin healing the incision.

    b. on both breasts as long as she is comfortable and the baby's mouth avoids the incision.

    c. only if she also offers other nourishment to her infant.

    d. only on the unaffected breast until the incision is entirely healed.

Discussion Questions

1. Describe at least five ways to treat a plugged duct.

2. What is a fibrocystic breast condition? Is it a contraindication to breastfeeding? Provide the rationale for your response.

3. What is an intraductal papilloma? How is it identified? What is its effect on lactation?

4. What factors seem to predispose women to develop mastitis? Discuss at least four factors and emphasize interactions among factors.

5. What is a nipple blister? How is it recognized? How should it be treated?

6. What is candidiasis? How is it identified? In what regions of the body can *Candida* lodge? In what members of the family can it be found?

7. What are common (although by no means universal) causes of lumps in the lactating breast?

8. What procedures are used to determine if breast lumps are cancerous or benign? Does breastfeeding need to be interrupted or terminated if such a procedure is to be performed?

9. Can breast cancer develop in breastfeeding women (or women who have breastfed)? Is it harmful for an infant to breastfeed if his mother has (or has had) breast cancer? Explain the rationale for your response.

10

Low Intake in the Breastfed Infant

Introduction

"Low intake" here refers not to some fixed volume of breastmilk but to the adequacy of intake as compared with the infant's needs. A baby whose weight gain is inadequate must be assessed in relation to his mother; either may be the independent cause of poor infant weight gain. Even so, their intimate interaction produces responses in each other that may exacerbate the infant's condition. Questions in this chapter will help you to assess your understanding of how to evaluate and manage the breastfeeding dyad when the infant's intake is inadequate.

IBLCE Disciplines

Information in this chapter applies to the following disciplines tested on the certification examination offered by the International Board of Lactation Consultant Examiners: B = Maternal and Infant Normal Physiology and Endocrinology; C = Maternal and Infant Normal Nutrition and Biochemistry; F = Maternal and Infant Pharmacology and Toxicology; K = Breastfeeding Equipment and Technology; L = Techniques; 3 = Perinatal; 4 = Prematurity; 5 = 0–2 days; 6 = 3–14 days; 12 = General Principles.

Multiple-Choice Questions

1. When a breastfed infant is not gaining normally, an LC or physician needs to examine
   a. the baby only.
   b. the mother only.
   c. the mother and baby.

2. Global growth standards released in 2006 by the World Health Organization, and based on the growth of healthy, predominantly breastfed infants around the world, will likely result in the greater prevalence of infants identified as all of the following *except*

   a. obese.

   b. overweight after 6 months.

   c. short for age.

   d. underweight during months 0–6.

3. A chief complaint about United States Centers for Disease Control standard infant growth charts—which are also used in many other countries—released in the year 2000 is that they are based on all of the following *except*

   a. data that began measurements at 2 months of infant age.

   b. infants principally fed formula.

   c. infants in the United States only.

   d. tracking infants longitudinally.

4. Infant weight loss in the first 3 days after birth is all of the following *except*

   a. associated with loss of fluid as circulating infant hormones increase.

   b. associated with loss of fluid as circulating maternal hormones decline.

   c. associated with small fluid intake from colostrum.

   d. experienced by most infants.

5. An infant is likely to lose more weight than the average range if his mother experienced any of the following *except*

   a. being markedly overweight.

   b. flat or inverted nipples.

   c. onset of lactogenesis II later than 72 hours.

   d. rapid labor (less than 8 hours).

6. The *most* important factor in a mother's continuing milk production is

   a. good positioning of the infant at the breast.

   b. removal of most of the milk in the breast at each feed.

   c. skin-to-skin contact with her infant.

   d. unlimited infant access to the breast.

7. In nearly all instances, milk production is related more closely to

   a. effective milk removal by the baby than maternal ability to synthesize milk.

   b. maternal ability to synthesize milk than effective removal of milk by the infant.

   c. maternal nutritional status than to size of the baby at birth.

   d. size of the baby at birth than to maternal nutritional status.

8. As compared with women of normal weight, overweight or obese women are more likely to have

   a. consistently larger volumes of colostrum.

   b. delayed onset of copious milk production.

   c. muted response to oxytocin.

   d. somewhat longer average duration of breastfeeding.

9. A neonatal weight loss in the range 7–9 percent should trigger what reaction?

   a. Add small water supplements to compensate for water loss.

   b. Evaluate mother and infant for adequate breastmilk transfer.

   c. None if baby is otherwise healthy; loss is within normal range.

   d. Physician should evaluate infant for possible health problems.

10. Return to birth weight is expected by day

    a. 8.

    b. 10.

    c. 12.

    d. 14.

11. As compared with the normally recommended daily weight gain, a weight gain of 20 grams per day in a 3-week-old infant is

    a. normal, if the baby regained birth weight on schedule.

    b. slightly above.

    c. slightly below.

    d. the minimum expected.

12. The average daily weight gain of fully breastfed infants is _____ grams per day for girls and _____ grams per day for boys.

    a. 25 / 31

    b. 31 / 33

    c. 34 / 40

    d. 40 / 40

13. If an infant is not gaining weight during his first month, one can also assume all of the following *except* that the

    a. baby is not removing milk effectively from the breast.

    b. mother's milk supply is declining.

    c. mother never had much milk to begin with.

    d. poor weight gain is more likely to be related to feeding inefficiency than to a medical problem.

14. Delayed onset of copious milk production has been associated with all of the following *except*

    a. excessive weight gain during pregnancy.

    b. flat or inverted nipples.

    c. insulin-dependent diabetes.

    d. very fair hair and skin.

15. Delayed onset of copious milk production is also associated with _____ during labor and delivery.

    a. a planned at-home stay

    b. excessive fatigue

    c. physical activity, such as walking or showering

    d. rapid progression of stage II labor

16. If birth edema related to maternal intravenous fluids during labor is not considered, infant weight loss greater than 10 percent in the first 72 hours most commonly is associated with
    a. colostrum as the only breast fluid in that interval.
    b. early milk production that is principally foremilk.
    c. excessive excretion of urine.
    d. letdown too rapid for the infant to take milk easily.

17. Infant weight loss greater than 10 percent in the first 72 hours is also associated with _____ infants, because they are likely to _____
    a. large / be placid and not cue to feed.
    b. large / have larger fat stores that diminish appetite for the first few days.
    c. small / have a small-breasted mother
    d. small / suckle more weakly.

18. A lactation consultant should suspect truly insufficient milk in the mother if all of the following are true *except*
    a. baby feeds appropriately.
    b. baby's weight gain is only about 35 grams per day.
    c. mother is motivated to continue breastfeeding.
    d. mother uses skilled assistance with breastfeeding.

19. An infant delivered at 35–37 weeks gestational age is apt to
    a. be jittery.
    b. be too sleepy to feed well.
    c. breastfeed about as easily as most term infants.
    d. clench his jaw or bite while nursing.

20. As compared with a healthy full-term newborn, an otherwise healthy infant born at 36 weeks gestation is _____ to feed poorly and become jaundiced.
    a. about as likely
    b. less likely
    c. much more likely
    d. very slightly more likely

21. As compared with a full-term breastfed infant, a breastfed infant born at 35–37 weeks is apt to be characterized by a
    a. higher rate of readmission to hospital.
    b. lower death rate in the first month.
    c. similar course of breastfeeding.
    d. similar rate of readmission to hospital.

22. Effective milk transfer in the healthy infant requires all of the following *except*
    a. gums well back on areola or breast.
    b. normal muscle tone.
    c. stomach-to-stomach nursing position.
    d. well-coordinated suck and swallow.

23. A weak suck in the infant may be associated with all of the following *except*
    a. maternal plugged ducts or mastitis.
    b. suck and swallow at irregular intervals.
    c. tonic bite.
    d. weight gain below reference standards.

24. Cow-milk allergy in a fully breastfed infant
    a. can be avoided if the mother consumes no fresh milk.
    b. has not been confirmed.
    c. is more apt in fact to be caused by an inhaled allergen.
    d. may be signaled by gastroesophageal reflux in the infant.

25. A baby who is quite plump despite being fussy at the breast and who has many thin or foamy stools likely has a mother who has
    a. a malabsorption problem.
    b. consumed too many carbonated beverages.
    c. passed her malabsorption problem on to her infant.
    d. very large volumes of foremilk.

26. Tongue-tie in an infant typically is associated with all of the following *except*
    a. abnormally high muscle tone.
    b. clenching or biting while feeding.
    c. indentation in the end of the baby's tongue.
    d. maternal sore nipples.

27. Clipping the frenulum under a tied tongue is
    a. a safe way to improve milk transfer in nearly all infants.
    b. necessary only if the frenulum appears to be particularly short or thick.
    c. rarely found to allow the baby's tongue to extend past his gum ridge.
    d. risky because of typical blood loss.

28. As compared with women who have normally protuberant nipples, women who have flat or inverted nipples have about _____ rate of delayed onset of copious milk production.
    a. half the
    b. the same
    c. twice the
    d. two and a half times the

29. The *most* effective way for a mother with flat or inverted nipples to breastfeed effectively is to
    a. assume that the neonate will pull out her nipples during feedings.
    b. stretch the nipple every day beginning in the second trimester.
    c. wear breast shells during pregnancy.
    d. work with a skilled lactation specialist to ensure that the neonate latches well.

30. Although nipple shields should be used with caution, thin silicone nipple shields may be useful for a time in all of the following situations *except* to

    a. avoid pumping the breasts between feedings.

    b. impede rapid flow of milk during letdown.

    c. permit a secure infant latch onto the breast.

    d. protect sore nipples.

31. The volume of milk produced can be reduced by all of the following *except*

    a. a subsequent conception during the breastfeeding interval.

    b. barrier contraceptives.

    c. fragments of placenta retained in the uterus.

    d. thyroid disorders.

32. Maternal smoking is associated with all of the following *except*

    a. decreased effectiveness of letdowns.

    b. larger milk volume.

    c. shorter total duration of breastfeeding.

    d. slower infant weight gain.

33. Alcohol consumption inhibits milk ejection

    a. but encourages infants to ingest more milk within 2 hours after maternal alcohol consumption.

    b. in direct relation to dose.

    c. in inverse relation to dose.

    d. once the plasma alcohol content exceeds some threshold.

34. As compared with women of normal weight consuming a nutritious diet, women who are under-weight or who consume a diet lacking in nutrients produce

    a. larger milk volumes, to make up for less-nutrient-dense milk.

    b. smaller milk volumes, because that is all their body stores will allow.

    c. smaller milk volumes, because that is all their diet will allow.

    d. typically about the same volume of milk.

35. Breast augmentation surgery is associated with increased risk of insufficient milk, because this surgery may be a marker for

    a. flat or inverted nipples that are hard for the baby to latch onto.

    b. lack of a full quota of milk-producing tissue.

    c. lack of real interest in breastfeeding.

    d. low concentrations of prolactin.

36. Women who are unable to nourish their infants at the breast because of "insufficient glandular development" typically have

    a. infants who latch and suckle poorly.

    b. low baseline prolactin concentrations.

    c. typical breast enlargement and tenderness during pregnancy.

    d. widely spaced, small, or tube-shaped breasts.

37. Underweight or poorly nourished women can *best* increase their milk supply by

    a. avoiding unneeded physical activity during the course of breastfeeding.

    b. improving overall nutrition during pregnancy.

    c. increasing calorie intake while breastfeeding.

    d. increasing fluid intake while breastfeeding.

38. A general rule for infant intake (in the first few months) is 150–200 ml per kilogram per day (ml/kg/day) of

    a. breastmilk.

    b. breastmilk, but about 20 percent more formula.

    c. either breastmilk or formula.

    d. formula, but about 20 percent more breastmilk.

39. A feeding-tube device works well for young infants who

    a. are weak or fatigue easily at the breast.

    b. coordinate sucking and breathing poorly at the breast.

    c. are normal but whose mother's milk supply is low.

    d. fall asleep easily at the breast.

40. When one test weighs an infant to determine his breastmilk intake, weighing

    a. at any one feeding is sufficient for calculating overall daily intake.

    b. gives an amount in grams that is about the same as the milliliters ingested.

    c. on an office (or grocery store) scale is sufficient.

    d. the normal, thriving infant regularly is recommended to reinforce the mother's observations.

Discussion Questions

1. What is tongue-tie? How do you identify it? If it is not treated, what are the consequences for breast-feeding? How is tongue-tie corrected?

2. What are the common consequences to breastfeeding of the following situations? What mechanism of action produces those consequences?

    • Pregnancy superimposed on lactation

    • Contraceptive pills begun early in lactation

    • Cigarette smoking

    • Hypothyroidism

    • Hyperthyroidism

    • Alcohol ingestion

3. What factors predispose a postpartum woman to delayed lactogenesis II? Describe four maternal factors and two infant factors.

4. What is the importance of listening for infant swallowing when one is evaluating a slow-gaining infant?

5. How might disorganized suckling in a newborn affect the establishment of breastfeeding? What might have caused this disorganization? What practices help to establish breastfeeding in the face of a disorganized suck?

6. What is the relation between poor infant weight gain and low maternal milk volumes? Describe conditions that might make the mother the independent variable. Describe conditions that might make the infant the independent variable.

7. What are the two most obvious indicators of inadequate breastmilk intake by an infant?

8. What is the difference between a slow-gaining baby and a failure-to-thrive baby? How do growth curves play into this diagnosis?

9. In the United States, from what populations were traditional growth curves (those of the National Center for Health Statistics) derived? Are these traditional growth curves adequate for assessing breastfed infants?

10. How were the new World Health Organization multicenter growth curves derived? Are they prescriptive or descriptive? What will be their effect in assessments of infant growth as compared with traditional growth curves?

11. During their first year, are breastfed babies underfed or are babies fed manufactured milks overfed? What is the rationale for your response? Do breastfed infants falter in growth around 3 or 4 months of age?

12. How does a mother's nutritional status during lactation affect her milk volumes?

13. How would you distinguish between the following infants, when all have their eyes closed while at the breast?
    • A satiated baby
    • A sleepy baby
    • A baby who is suffering from failure to thrive

14. Describe at least four infant health conditions that can result in failure to thrive. How can the condition be recognized? How can breastfeeding still be maintained?

15. What is the role of nighttime feedings in promoting adequate infant weight gain? What is the physiological basis for this role?

Jaundice and the Breastfed Baby

Introduction

Jaundice is the great conundrum of early breastfeeding: How can the perfect infant food sometimes lead to a possibly life-threatening illness in the neonate? The lactation consultant should be able to distinguish between common physiologic jaundice, nonbreastfeeding jaundice, and pathologic jaundice and understand how each is managed. Questions in this chapter will help you to assess your understanding of this body of information and how it applies to professional practice.

IBLCE Disciplines

Information in this chapter applies to the following disciplines tested on the certification examination offered by the International Board of Lactation Consultant Examiners: B = Maternal and Infant Normal Physiology and Endocrinology; C = Maternal and Infant Normal Nutrition and Biochemistry; D = Maternal and Infant Immunology and Infectious Disease; E = Maternal and Infant Pathology; F = Maternal and Infant Pharmacology and Toxicology; 3 = Perinatal; 4 = Prematurity; 5 = 0–2 days; 6 = 3–14 days; 7 = 15–28 days.

Multiple-Choice Questions

1. Jaundice refers to progressive yellowing of a newborn's

   a. palms of hands, then soles of feet.

   b. sclerae and skin.

   c. stools.

   d. urine.

2. Physiologic jaundice is a condition that develops chiefly in infants who
   a. are born at term and are healthy—about two-thirds of all newborns.
   b. are born to mothers who lacked good prenatal care.
   c. are placid and do not cue to feed.
   d. have an underlying medical problem, such as malabsorption.

3. In the young infant, physiologic jaundice is caused by normal mild elevation of
   a. conjugated (bound) bilirubin in plasma.
   b. conjugated (bound) bilirubin in stools.
   c. unconjugated (unbound) bilirubin in breastmilk.
   d. unconjugated (unbound) bilirubin in plasma.

4. Physiologic jaundice in full-term, formula-fed newborns typically resolves
   a. by day 7.
   b. by day 21.
   c. after bilirubin concentrations elevate to normal values.
   d. after biliverdin concentrations drop to normal values.

5. In healthy, adequately fed newborns during the first 5 days of life, serum bilirubin concentrations typically are about _____ in breastfed infants as compared with formula-fed infants.
   a. 18 percent higher
   b. 18 percent lower
   c. 30 percent lower
   d. the same

6. A healthy, thriving, 4-week-old breastfed infant who has visibly jaundiced skin should be
   a. fed at the breast on demand.
   b. weaned from the breast and fed formula to resolve the jaundice.
   c. seen by a physician to determine if the infant has an underlying medical problem.
   d. supplemented with formula to resolve the jaundice.

7. Breastmilk jaundice results from a factor in breastmilk that promotes a(an) _____ in the _____.
   a. decrease / production of plasma proteins.
   b. increase / intestinal absorption of bilirubin.
   c. increase / production of bilirubin.
   d. increase / production of biliverdin, which is metabolized to bilirubin.

8. In 4-day-old well-fed neonates, serum concentration of bilirubin is
   a. a little higher in breastfed infants.
   b. about the same in breastfed and formula-fed infants.
   c. much higher in adequately breastfeed infants.
   d. much higher in formula-fed infants.

9. It is sometimes recommended that mothers of jaundiced infants interrupt breastfeeding for 1 or 2 days to reduce serum bilirubin concentration to
    a. a value that the infant then maintains.
    b. a value that will rebound, but not as high as before.
    c. allow the breast to slightly diminish milk volume, thus requiring the infant to expend less energy digesting milk.
    d. allow the baby to spend fewer minutes per day feeding and thus conserve energy.

10. All of the following statements are true *except*
    a. bilirubin is an effective antioxidant.
    b. newborns lack antioxidants.
    c. antioxidants present in more than trace amounts are cause for concern.
    d. bilirubin may help protect the infant.

11. As compared with the norm, bilirubin concentration of about 16 milligrams per deciliter in a jaundiced infant suggests _____ bilirubin production or _____ bilirubin excretion.
    a. faster / faster
    b. faster / slower
    c. slower / faster
    d. slower / slower

12. Elevated bilirubin concentration in the first 3 or so days of life may reflect
    a. formula supplement before lactogenesis II.
    b. excessive intake of foremilk.
    c. high urine output.
    d. retention of fecal material.

13. The production of bilirubin from dead red blood cells passes through intermediate stages that produce all of the following *except*
    a. hemoglobin.
    b. heme.
    c. biliverdin.
    d. carbon dioxide.

14. The plasma concentration of bilirubin in neonates, as compared with that of adults, is
    a. about the same.
    b. difficult to specify because it varies so greatly.
    c. higher.
    d. lower.

15. Factors contributing to physiologic neonatal jaundice include all of the following *except*
    a. large volume of fetal red blood cells.
    b. relatively large blood volume, augmented at birth by cord blood.
    c. relatively short life of fetal red blood cells.
    d. sharp decrease in rate of destruction of fetal red blood cells after birth.

16. The bilirubin molecule that causes jaundice is eventually removed from circulation by being compartmentalized principally in an infant's
    a. intestinal wall.
    b. liver.
    c. stools.
    d. urine.

17. Bilirubin that may pose the larger health threat to the infant is known as all of the following *except*
    a. direct-reacting bilirubin.
    b. indirect-reacting bilirubin.
    c. insoluble bilirubin.
    d. unconjugated bilirubin.

18. Physiologic jaundice of the newborn is caused by
    a. circulation of more bilirubin than the liver can remove from circulation.
    b. infrequent urination before lactogenesis II is established.
    c. resorption of occult blood originating in the intestinal wall.
    d. the neonate's mild autoimmune reaction to heme released from his own degraded red blood cells.

19. An enzyme (beta-glucuronidase) that is abundant in the infant's intestinal wall acts to
    a. make insoluble bilirubin soluble, and thus able to reenter the infant's circulation.
    b. make soluble bilirubin insoluble, and thus able to reenter the infant's circulation.
    c. remove proteins that otherwise promote recirculation of bilirubin.
    d. sequester bilirubin by binding to it.

20. As an infant's plasma concentration of bilirubin increases, yellowish tinting of the skin progresses from
    a. eyes and head to foot.
    b. fingertips and toes to torso.
    c. soles of feet to head.
    d. torso to extremities.

21. The *best* way to determine an infant's plasma concentration of bilirubin is by
    a. close, regular inspection of the infant's skin.
    b. use of a transcutaneous measurement device.
    c. serum measurement plotted on a nomogram.
    d. test weighing the infant; milk intake is inversely related to bilirubin concentration.

22. In formula-fed infants, plasma bilirubin concentration typically peaks at a higher value in infants of _____ ancestry.
    a. Asian
    b. Caucasian
    c. Hispanic
    d. Middle Eastern

23. Breastmilk jaundice typically is seen in infants with all of the following characteristics *except*

    a. conjugated bilirubin greater than 10 percent of total bilirubin.

    b. healthy and gaining weight normally.

    c. stools distinctly yellow.

    d. conjugated bilirubin less than 10 percent of total bilirubin.

24. Breastmilk jaundice is *best* considered a(an)

    a. early sign of a tendency to food allergy.

    b. normal physiologic phenomenon.

    c. sign of an underlying abnormality in digestion of breastmilk.

    d. treatable illness in the infant.

25. Breastmilk jaundice results from increased _____ after lactogenesis II is well established.

    a. destruction of red blood cells

    b. intestinal absorption of bilirubin

    c. rate of transport of conjugated bilirubin into the liver

    d. transport of unconjugated bilirubin out of the liver

26. Starvation jaundice typically manifests

    a. during the first 24 hours postpartum when little colostrum is available.

    b. in infants whose mothers ingest large quantities of dairy foods.

    c. only after copious milk production is established.

    d. prior to establishment of copious milk production.

27. After _____ adults fast for 24 hours, _____.

    a. healthy / a yellowish color tinges the whites of the eyes.

    b. healthy / normal adult bilirubin concentration doubles.

    c. debilitated / normal adult bilirubin concentration doubles.

    d. Asian and Native American / a yellowish color tinges the whites of the eyes.

28. An apparently healthy neonate who is fed only at the breast but who, by a 48-hour discharge time, does not feed well should be _____, where _____.

    a. released home / mother and thus baby will be more relaxed, and baby will feed better.

    b. released home / the mother can adhere to scheduled feedings more easily.

    c. retained in hospital / possible sepsis can be fully investigated.

    d. retained in hospital / skilled assistance with breastfeeding is available.

29. When severe jaundice develops in a poorly breastfeeding neonate, the *best* response to ensure the baby's health is to

    a. avoid possible allergic response to manufactured milk by continuing to feed only at the breast.

    b. for a limited time supplement the infant while skilled assistance helps to resolve the breastfeeding problem.

    c. promptly lower the baby's bilirubin concentration by weaning the baby to formula.

    d. supplement the infant, but with water only to ensure good hydration.

30. Neonates in whom jaundice developed secondary to poor breastmilk intake ("starvation jaundice") are later at _____ risk for very high bilirubin concentrations once lactogenesis II has occurred, because _____.

    a. lesser / barrier mucosa in the intestines has had time to mature.

    b. lesser / the two cancel out each other.

    c. greater / effects of the two are additive.

    d. no greater risk / the two operate in different infant compartments.

31. The form of bilirubin that stains brain tissue is

    a. a biliverdin molecule.

    b. a bilirubin stereoisomer.

    c. conjugated.

    d. unconjugated.

32. Initially, a neonatal infection and bilirubin staining of brain tissue (kernicterus) may both present as all of the following *except*

    a. body temperature lower than 97°C.

    b. lethargy.

    c. poor feeding.

    d. respiratory difficulty.

33. Survivors of severe stages of kernicterus are *least* likely to experience

    a. cerebral palsy.

    b. deafness.

    c. impaired intellectual function.

    d. inability to swallow.

34. Which of the following factors is *least* likely to promote hyperbilirubinemia?

    a. Breastfeeding

    b. Cephalhematoma

    c. Late-preterm gestational age at birth

    d. Respiratory distress syndrome

35. Kernicterus is promoted by all of the following *except*

    a. decreased concentration of unbound serum albumin.

    b. decreased enterohepatic circulation of bilirubin.

    c. degradation of red blood cells.

    d. increased permeability of the blood-brain barrier.

36. Biliverdin, one product of the degradation of red blood cells, is

    a. fat soluble.

    b. produced in amounts equimolar with CO_2 and iron.

    c. reduced to form unconjugated bilirubin.

    d. toxic to the infant in more than trace amounts.

37. To accelerate the decline of bilirubin concentration, a breastfed infant being treated for jaundice by phototherapy should be

    a. breastfed at least 8 times per day for as much as 30 minutes each to maintain nutritive intake.

    b. fed by bottle to maximize the amount of time spent under the phototherapy lights.

    c. fed intravenously to ensure that he stays hydrated.

    d. offered only water by mouth during the first 24 hours of treatment.

38. The effectiveness of phototherapy is based on its ability to _____, thus increasing excretion.

    a. alter unbound bilirubin into a form that requires no further processing before it can be excreted

    b. alter unbound water-soluble bilirubin to fat-soluble bilirubin

    c. decrease the abundance of glucuronic acid, which inhibits conjugation of bilirubin

    d. increase the number of transport proteins that move bilirubin through the liver

Discussion Questions

1. How will answers to each of the following questions help you evaluate an infant's risk of early-onset infant jaundice?

   • How many times is the infant put to breast in 24 hours?

   • How are feedings distributed during any 24-hour period?

   • How effectively is the baby suckling?

   • How often does the baby stool? What do the stools look like?

   • Besides breastmilk, what other fluids is the baby being given?

   • What is baby's change in weight since birth?

   • Are the mother's nipples comfortable?

   • How does ethnicity affect normal serum bilirubin levels in newborn infants?

   • How do these differences affect the care given those infants?

2. Should breastfeeding be interrupted for a day or two to reduce serum bilirubin levels in infants being treated under bilirubin lights?

3. Is it ever reasonable to briefly interrupt use of bilirubin lights in order to feed or comfort the treated infant?

4. How can the following be distinguished?

   • Normal early jaundice

   • Breastmilk jaundice

   • Pathological jaundice

5. Is there any possible benefit to modestly elevated bilirubin concentrations in neonates?

6. Why are infants fed manufactured milks less likely to receive a diagnosis of jaundice in the first few days of life? Is this fact sufficient justification for feeding artificial milks during this interval?

7. How might hospital routines influence the likelihood of severe hyperbilirubinemia in an infant?

   • Use of analgesia or anesthesia

   • Type of infant feeding

Breast Pumps
and Other Technologies

Introduction

Sometimes this most natural way to feed and mother an infant benefits from some technological help. Babies are the best breastmilk extractor, but babies are not always available when milk needs to be removed. Specialized devices protect the breast and increasingly are used to obtain milk and sustain the milk-producing capacity of the breast in both short-term and long-term situations. Lactation consultants should understand the principles upon which various types of pumps work and how to fit a pump to the mother for optimal performance. Questions in this chapter will help you to assess your understanding of this body of information and how it applies to professional practice.

IBLCE Disciplines

Information in this chapter applies to the following disciplines tested on the certification examination offered by the International Board of Lactation Consultant Examiners: B = Maternal and Infant Normal Physiology and Endocrinology; E = Maternal and Infant Pathology; G = Psychology, Sociology, and Anthropology; K = Breastfeeding Equipment and Technology; L = Techniques; 3 = Perinatal; 4 = Prematurity; 5 = 0–2 days; 6 = 3–14 days; 7 = 15–28 days; 12 = General Principles.

Multiple-Choice Questions

1. In order to increase the amount of milk obtained by pumping, a mother should _____ in order to _____.

   a. apply cool compresses on the breasts before pumping / help milk alveoli contract.

   b. exercise vigorously for a few minutes before pumping / promote good blood flow in the breast.

   c. massage the breasts while pumping / increase intramammary pressure.

   d. pump for at least 5 minutes after the last milk is obtained / ensure that all milk available has been taken.

2. Mothers who feel a milk-ejection reflex find that it
   a. is a single event at the beginning of a feeding.
   b. is elicited more rapidly by a hospital-grade electric pump than by a baby.
   c. requires tactile stimulation of the nipple.
   d. takes about a minute to occur after a baby first begins to suckle.

3. Massaging the breasts during a pumping may do all of the following *except*
   a. increase fat content of the milk.
   b. increase milk yield.
   c. increase nipple pain.
   d. increase plasma oxytocin concentration.

4. The oxytocin release that results in the milk ejection reflex
   a. comes in several brief bursts only at the beginning of a feeding.
   b. increases the diameter of milk ducts by about 25 percent.
   c. is enhanced by massaging the breasts while nursing or pumping.
   d. lengthens the milk ducts.

5. When is a mother most likely to pump the most milk at a single pumping session?
   a. After any interval greater than 3 hours when no milk has been removed
   b. Before bed
   c. Noon to 6:00 pm
   d. Shortly after awakening in the morning

6. The *best* time for a healthy mother with a newborn unable to nurse to begin pumping her breasts is no later than _____ hours postpartum.
   a. 24
   b. 12
   c. 6
   d. 2

7. For optimal response to a breast pump, a mother should elicit the milk-ejection reflex
   a. after she has pumped about 2 minutes.
   b. before she begins pumping.
   c. immediately after she begins pumping.
   d. when milk begins to flow.

8. Pumping the breasts for several minutes after milk stops flowing or dripping rapidly
   a. ensures that nipples will remain everted.
   b. markedly increases future milk supply.
   c. may damage breast tissue.
   d. promotes further letdowns at that pumping episode.

9. Prolactin concentration in the blood varies in all of the following ways *except*
    a. by 6 months postpartum it rises about 10-20% with the stimulus of suckling.
    b. drops to baseline by about 6 months postpartum.
    c. in the early weeks it typically doubles with the stimulus of suckling.
    d. it rises during pregnancy from about 10 to 200 nanograms/ml.

10. In initiating and sustaining breastmilk production, prolactin
    a. acts to increase milk production when mother's supply is low.
    b. acts to decrease milk production when baby takes less milk than mother secretes.
    c. binds less effectively to receptors in mammary tissue as lactation progresses.
    d. permits, but does not regulate, milk production.

11. The rapid increase in prolactin concentration initiated by suckling is _____ the mother's ambient plasma prolactin concentration.
    a. added to
    b. additive during normal sleeping hours but does not affect it during normal waking hours
    c. not affected by
    d. subtracted from

12. Removal of milk from the breasts by a nursing baby or by a pump is a prerequisite for
    a. galactopoiesis.
    b. involution.
    c. lactogenesis I.
    d. lactogenesis II.

13. Few attempts to put a baby to breast or to pump during the first three days postpartum may contribute to all of the following *except*
    a. delay in lactogenesis II.
    b. fewer than optimal prolactin receptors in the breast.
    c. increased initial milk volume when lactogenesis II does occur.
    d. low milk supply.

14. The best action for a mother with painfully engorged breasts is to
    a. apply ice packs to her breasts for 20 minutes of each hour.
    b. bind her breasts.
    c. pump or hand express milk as needed to stay comfortable.
    d. restrict fluid intake.

15. As compared with mothers who have large breasts, mothers with small breasts typically
    a. are less likely to pump sufficient milk for a nonnursing infant.
    b. have lower fat content in hindmilk.
    c. need to pump more frequently per day to remain comfortable.
    d. take longer to achieve the milk-ejection reflex.

16. As compared with the left breast, the right breast tends to
    a. be slightly cooler.
    b. produce more milk.
    c. receive a smaller blood supply.
    d. take longer to elicit a milk-ejection reflex.

17. After a milk-ejection response, all of the following happen *except*
    a. about 1 ounce (about 30 ml) of milk transfers to a healthy nursing infant.
    b. if it is the first ejection of a nursing session, it provides the largest volume of milk.
    c. milk ducts remain dilated for about 1 to 3 minutes.
    d. the rate of milk removal is stable for the duration of the feeding.

18. Women with the largest increase in ductal diameter during a milk-ejection reflex
    a. needed to pump longer in order to take all available milk.
    b. pumped larger volumes of milk.
    c. pumped smaller volumes of milk.
    d. subsequently secreted milk more slowly.

19. The *principal* mechanism by which a breast pump causes milk to flow from the breast is by
    a. creating a pressure gradient, down which milk flows.
    b. mechanical kneading of the breast that squeezes out the milk, like toothpaste from a tube.
    c. mimicking the sensations produced by a suckling infant, which stimulate oxytocin release.
    d. suction, like sucking on a straw.

20. The vacuum that an infant applies to the breast
    a. is a constant value.
    b. both stretches the nipple and increases its diameter.
    c. is the sole process that draws milk from the nipple.
    d. rises and falls but maintains a basal value sufficient to maintain latch.

21. During suckling at the breast, an infant typically does all of the following *except*
    a. apply suction during about half of each suck cycle.
    b. complete about 40–120 suck cycles per minute.
    c. create a suction in the range of −50 to −150 millimeters of mercury.
    d. squeeze milk into his mouth solely by compressing breast tissue against the roof of his mouth.

22. The highest spike in plasma prolactin concentration produced by something other than a baby is
    a. hand expression of one breast at a time.
    b. manual pumping of one breast at a time.
    c. using a hospital-grade electric pump on both breasts simultaneously.
    d. using a hospital-grade electric pump on one breast at a time.

23. The *best* manual pumps have all of the following features *except* a(an)

    a. adjustable vacuum settings.

    b. collection bottle to accumulate milk.

    c. device that automatically interrupts the vacuum at a specified intensity.

    d. outer cylinder to accumulate milk.

24. Hospital-grade electric pumps typically cycle suction on and off at a rate that _____ the typical rate of an infant, to _____.

    a. is lower than / reduce the likelihood of nipple damage.

    b. is somewhat higher than / optimize milk yield.

    c. is similar to / mimic the action of an infant

    d. varies / mimic natural infant variation.

25. During pumping, the nipples typically will

    a. be less apt to bind in the pump's breast flange as pumping proceeds.

    b. lengthen and decrease in diameter, similar to changes during nursing.

    c. shorten but increase in diameter.

    d. swell in response to the vacuum.

26. As compared with a healthy, full-term infant, a compromised preterm infant will likely tolerate a _____ concentration of nonpathogenic bacteria and a _____ concentration of pathogenic bacteria.

    a. higher / lower

    b. lower / higher

    c. lower / zero

    d. zero / lower

27. A compromised newborn who is fed breastmilk will receive the least-altered milk if he is fed in all the following ways *except*

    a. directly at the breast insofar as is possible.

    b. pasteurized rather than refrigerated milk.

    c. refrigerated rather than thawed frozen milk.

    d. small bolus feedings rather than continuous feedings.

28. Freshly pumped breastmilk

    a. contains bacteria only if it has been contaminated by poor pumping technique.

    b. contains bacteria only if the mother herself has a bacterial infection.

    c. is always sterile.

    d. usually contains only nonpathogenic bacteria.

29. Most pumps are adequately cleaned by all of the following procedures *except*

    a. drying in air.

    b. rinsing thoroughly.

    c. swabbing surfaces lightly with an abrasive.

    d. washing in hot, soapy water.

30. To make the best use of breast pump, a mother needs to
    a. develop outside activities that offer relief from the demands of a newborn.
    b. know how much milk she should collect at each pumping session.
    c. receive clear instructions and emotional support.
    d. take a day off from pumping from time to time.

31. In the United States, breast pumps are regulated by the
    a. department of health in each state.
    b. U.S. Department of Health, Education, and Welfare.
    c. U.S. Food and Drug Administration.
    d. U.S. National Institutes of Health.

32. To avoid injury, a mother who uses a hand-operated cylinder breast pump should position her "pumping" arm as follows *except* for
    a. elbow next to body.
    b. forearm turned up (little finger toward the midline).
    c. shoulder raised toward ear.
    d. wrist slightly flexed.

33. To increase the quantity of milk collected, the *best* action for a mother who expresses only small amounts of milk is to
    a. drink additional water during the day.
    b. elicit a milk-ejection reflex before beginning to pump.
    c. use a breast flange that comfortably accommodates her breast and nipple.
    d. use a pump with a manually controlled vacuum setting.

34. Pumping practices that reduce the likelihood of sore nipples are using all of the following *except*
    a. a breast flange that accommodates the nipple at the end of pumping.
    b. a breast flange that accommodates the nipple at the outset of pumping.
    c. the lowest vacuum that obtains milk.
    d. application of vacuum only after the milk-ejection reflex has been stimulated.

35. The largest release of milk during a single breastfeeding or pumping takes place
    a. in the 3 or 4 minutes after first milk ejection.
    b. at a point in the feeding or pumping that changes from session to session and probably is related to mother's emotional state.
    c. in the first milk-ejection episode.
    d. in the interval in which hindmilk is released.

36. As the course of breastfeeding or pumping lengthens, the milk-ejection reflex is triggered more
    a. quickly by a baby but more slowly by a pump.
    b. quickly by both baby and pump.
    c. slowly by both baby and pump.
    d. slowly by the baby but more quickly by the pump.

37. When a baby is properly positioned over a nipple shield, the baby's lips should be
    a. firmly adhered to the flat flange of the shield.
    b. on the shaft of the nipple shield.
    c. puckered or turned in.
    d. resting loosely on the flange.

38. A mother who has *Candida* on her areola should best clean nipple shields after a feeding by
    a. boiling for 20 minutes.
    b. rinsing in warm water and air drying.
    c. washing in hot, soapy water.
    d. washing in hot, soapy water with chlorine bleach.

39. The best action for a lactation consultant who recommends that a mother use a nipple shield is to
    a. document the recommendation, reasons for it, and instructions given to mother.
    b. explain to the mother risks and benefits of use of a nipple shield.
    c. instruct the mother in proper use of the nipple shield.
    d. send documentation of nipple shield recommendation to the mother's primary healthcare provider.

40. Breast shells are *best* used to
    a. catch milk leaked between feedings that can be stored for later use.
    b. collect milk that drips from one breast while the other is being nursed or pumped.
    c. evert flat or retracted nipples postpartum.
    d. protect a nipple inflamed with *Candida*.

41. Nipple shields can be useful temporary aids that help provide all of the following *except*
    a. compensation for weak infant suction.
    b. correction of low milk supply.
    c. oral stimulation of the infant's mouth.
    d. stability of nipple shape during the resting phase of the suckling cycle.

42. Use of a nipple shield may be indicated in all of the following situations *except* when baby has a
    a. large mouth and mother's nipple and areola are small.
    b. preference for artificial nipples.
    c. strongly recessed chin.
    d. very high muscle tone.

43. For a baby to use a feeding-tube device effectively, the baby
    a. need not be able to latch but must be able to suckle to some degree.
    b. need not be able to protect his airway because milk does not leak from the device.
    c. should be able to latch onto the breast and suckle to some degree.
    d. should have ample buccal pads.

Discussion Questions

1. In what situations might you consider recommending a nipple shield? In what situations would another alternative be better? What are those alternatives?

2. Should a mother always pump using the maximum negative pressure (suction) that a pump will generate? Why or why not? If not, how should she determine the degree of suction to use?

3. What is finger-feeding? When is it appropriate to use? Are there any risks involved in its use?

4. What are the phases of a breast pump cycle? How is each related to the phases of normal infant suckle?

5. Review the instructions accompanying two breast pump kits. Identify information that
   - is accurate.
   - is confusing.
   - improperly describes the lactation process.

6. How will your recommendations deal with inaccurate information in these or similar breast-pump kits?

Breastfeeding the Premature Infant

Introduction

The maternal body is to a degree primed to provide milk for preterm infants, and mother and baby receive physiological and emotional benefits from the act of breastfeeding that far exceed benefits received from the feeding of manufactured milks. Yet mothers of premature infants are among the least likely to breastfeed. Lactation consultants must understand how to help mothers bring in and maintain a milk supply in the absence of a vigorously nursing infant and how to help the infant maximize his breastmilk intake when he does come to the breast. Questions in this chapter will help you to assess your understanding of this body of information and how it applies to professional practice.

IBLCE Disciplines

Information in this chapter applies to the following disciplines tested on the certification examination offered by the International Board of Lactation Consultant Examiners: E = Maternal and Infant Pathology; F = Maternal and Infant Pharmacology and Toxicology; G = Psychology, Sociology, and Anthropology; K = Breastfeeding Equipment and Technology; L = Techniques; 4 = Prematurity; 12 = General Principles.

Multiple-Choice Questions

1. To provide her preterm infant with a health benefit, a mother should provide breastmilk for at least
   a. 1 month.
   b. one enteral feeding.
   c. until her milk comes in.
   d. until her milk fully matures (about day 14 postpartum).

2. Preterm mothers' milk typically is not able to sustain optimal
   a. bone mineralization.
   b. increase in head circumference.
   c. metabolic activity.
   d. weight gain.

3. The currently preferred feeding for younger premature infants is breastmilk that is
   a. fortified with calcium and phosphorus.
   b. fresh and unmodified.
   c. frozen and then thawed.
   d. refrigerated.

4. Published studies of mothers' feelings about having breastfed their hospitalized preterm infant show that the mothers felt that
   a. breastfeeding a premature infant was unpleasant.
   b. pumping breastmilk was inconvenient.
   c. the infant preferred being fed breastmilk by bottle to being fed at the breast.
   d. they gave their infant a good start in life.

5. Healthcare providers should talk about the benefits of breastfeeding preterm infants with _____ mothers who deliver preterm infants _____.
   a. all / and who ask about breastfeeding their preterm infant.
   b. all / whether they seem interested or not.
   c. only those / and who intend to breastfeed.
   d. only those / and who are undecided about breastfeeding.

6. Data gathered around the world show that mothers of preterm infants breastfeed at a rate that is
   a. about the same as the general population.
   b. higher than that of the general population.
   c. lower in industrialized nations but higher in developing nations.
   d. lower than that of the general population.

7. Counseling mothers of preterm infants about the benefits of breastfeeding _____ the initiation of breastfeeding _____.
   a. increased / but also increased maternal stress.
   b. increased / but only among those who had intended to breastfeed.
   c. increased / regardless of how the mother had intended to feed her infant.
   d. neither increased nor decreased / among mothers of preterm infants.

8. If a mother of a newly delivered preterm infant is reluctant to begin expressing breastmilk, a lactation consultant should tell her all of the following *except* that
   a. any amount of colostrum will benefit her infant more than formula.
   b. if she doesn't start pumping now it will be much harder to do so later.
   c. she can discontinue expressing milk at any time.
   d. staff will help her discontinue pumping.

9. During the first 10 days postpartum, the mother of a premature infant should pump her breasts _____ in order to _____.

   a. at least 8 times in 24 hours / bring in as good a milk supply as she can.

   b. at least 8 times in 24 hours / get accustomed to the frequency that her baby will feed once he is home.

   c. at least 8 times in 24 hours / stimulate lengthening of lactiferous ducts while lactogenic hormones are present in high concentration.

   d. just to comfort / regain her strength and spend time with her infant.

10. If expressed breastmilk is not stirred before being decanted into storage containers, the fat-rich portion of milk will be _____ the collection bottle, because the fat molecules _____.

    a. distributed evenly throughout / are more or less in equilibrium with other milk components.

    b. layered at the bottom of / are concentrated in the first milk expressed.

    c. layered at the bottom of / sink.

    d. layered at the top of / rise.

11. To collect a container of breastmilk with the highest calorie count possible, a mother should pump

    a. late in the evening and keep that milk separate from others.

    b. only until the initial letdown has passed, but do so three or four times an hour.

    c. until the milk begins to drip, then stop.

    d. until the milk entirely stops dripping.

12. Allowing mothers of hospitalized newborns to pump milk at their infant's bedside promotes all of the following *except*

    a. more-frequent visits to the hospitalized infant.

    b. increased stress for the mother.

    c. looking at or touching her infant during pumping, which helps a mother pump more milk.

    d. hospital staff's belief that providing mother's milk to the infant is important.

13. To be able to fully breastfeed her premature infant at the time he is ready for discharge, most mothers should produce at least _____ ml of breastmilk per day.

    a. 350

    b. 500

    c. 650

    d. 800

14. A mother who intends to fully breastfeed her premature infant, and who on day 14 postpartum is producing about 300 milliliters of milk per day, should

    a. be complimented for exceeding the volume of milk normally recommended for that point in time.

    b. more than double that amount of milk by the time her infant is discharged.

    c. pump according to a different routine to increase her milk supply.

    d. plan on combining breastfeeds with formula feeds.

15. A mother who pumps about 800 ml of milk per day for her small, 14-day-old preterm infant has

    a. a milk supply large enough to withstand substantial decline if her infant is hospitalized for many weeks.

    b. an oversupply of milk owing to poor hormonal regulation.

    c. an unnecessarily large milk supply in comparison with the small volumes consumed by her infant.

    d. fewer alveolar cells than mothers who pump lesser volumes.

16. Mothers with large milk-storage capacity synthesize milk _____ even when pumping sessions are _____.

    a. at a fairly consistent rate / further apart.

    b. more rapidly / more closely spaced.

    c. more slowly / further apart.

    d. more slowly / more closely spaced.

17. To calculate the rate of milk synthesis (milliliters per hour) prior to any one pumping session, measure the volume of milk collected at that session and

    a. add that volume to the volume of the previous session and divide by the number of hours between the two sessions.

    b. divide by the number of hours since the previous session.

    c. multiply by the number of hours since the previous session.

    d. subtract it from the volume of the subsequent session.

18. Before suggesting ways to increase a mother's milk supply, a lactation consultant should obtain information about all of the following *except*

    a. extended bed rest before this baby's birth.

    b. previous breastfeeding experience.

    c. sleep habits before she became pregnant.

    d. thyroid conditions and fertility concerns.

19. During the second month of milk expression, milk volumes pumped by most mothers of hospitalized premature infants _____ because _____.

    a. decrease / the mother's body conserves maternal energy for caring for her infant.

    b. decrease / the pump does not provide optimal stimulation of hormones that regulate milk production.

    c. increase / the rate of milk synthesis generally increases with time.

    d. remain more or less at the same level achieved about 2 weeks postpartum / of the hormonal support provided by galactopoesis.

20. Skin-to-skin ("kangaroo") care can be safely begun with infants

    a. once they remain stable in their cribs.

    b. only after they weigh at least 4 pounds and have no major medical problems.

    c. only after they weigh at least 4 pounds, regardless of other medical problems.

    d. who are very small, even if ventilated.

21. Freshly pumped mother's milk is

    a. sterile.

    b. sterile unless the mother's pumping technique is poor or equipment is contaminated.

    c. usually inoculated only with skin flora.

    d. usually inoculated with skin flora and pathogenic bacteria.

22. All of the following are true *except*

    a. freeze milk that will not be used within 48 hours of collection, but not until close to the 48-hour deadline.

    b. immediately freeze milk that will not be used within 48 hours of collection.

    c. refrigerate milk that will be fed between 1 and 48 hours of collection.

    d. use fresh, room-temperature expressed milk within 1 hour of collection.

23. Refrigerated or frozen mother's milk should be warmed before feeding by

    a. gradual heating for about 30 minutes to about body temperature.

    b. gradual heating for more than an hour to slightly more than body temperature to mimic the slightly higher temperature of the breast.

    c. rapid heating in a microwave oven to retain maximum nutrients.

    d. rapid heating in a microwave oven to retain maximal immunologic factors.

24. As compared with chilled or frozen breastmilk, fresh breastmilk better helps an infant

    a. form blood clots.

    b. grow in length.

    c. resist infection.

    d. resolve nonbreastmilk jaundice.

25. As compared with formula-fed premature infants, human-milk-fed premature infants typically tolerate a _____ volume of milk because _____.

    a. larger / human milk's fats are more easily digested than fats in formula.

    b. larger / human milk's whey:casein ratio allows it to leave the stomach more rapidly than formula.

    c. similar / human-milk feedings typically are fortified with calcium and phosphorus, so they digest at about the same rate as formula.

    d. smaller / otherwise the small intestine becomes distended, predisposing the infant to necrotizing enterocolitis.

26. All of the following statements about hindmilk are true *except* that hindmilk

    a. accelerates infant weight gain.

    b. contains a higher percentage of calories than foremilk or "average" milk.

    c. contains a higher percentage of fat than foremilk or "average" milk.

    d. precludes the need for breastmilk fortifiers.

27. Human milk fed to a premature infant by gavage should be administered by _____ gavage in order to _____
    a. continuous / avoid exceeding the capacity of the infant's stomach.
    b. continuous / encourage a stable concentration of blood glucose.
    c. intermittent bolus / to help regulate quiet alert states.
    d. slow intermittent bolus / to minimize loss of fats to that adhere to the gavage tube.

28. Lipid-soluble medications used by a breastfeeding mother are composed of molecules that generally are
    a. concentrated in hindmilk.
    b. concentrated in foremilk.
    c. of too short a half-life to be of concern.
    d. too large to pass into breastmilk.

29. Transmission of viral infections through breastmilk to the recipient infant is
    a. eliminated if the breastmilk is frozen and then thawed before feeding.
    b. not a concern, because viruses have not been documented to appear in breastmilk.
    c. not a concern, because viruses typically are destroyed in the infant stomach.
    d. thought to be less of a risk for the infant who receives only breastmilk feedings.

30. Nonnutritive sucking by an infant at his mother's breast tends to do all of the following *except*
    a. accustom the infant to the taste and smell of his mother's breastmilk.
    b. decrease infant physiologic stability.
    c. increase maternal yield of pumped milk.
    d. provide the infant with a gentle experience in his mouth.

31. As compared with premature infants fed by bottle, preterm infants fed at the breast typically do all of the following *except*
    a. breathe irregularly a smaller portion of the time.
    b. have a less-stable body temperature.
    c. have more stable oxygenation.
    d. ingest a larger volume of milk.

32. The *best* indicator that a premature infant is ready to feed at the breast is that the infant can
    a. consume full feedings by bottle.
    b. coordinate, to some extent, suck, swallow, and breathe.
    c. reliably maintain his body temperature.
    d. stay awake for a full feeding.

33. The *best* practice when beginning breastfeeds with a less-mature premature infant is for the mother to _____ in order to _____

    a. initiate letdown before putting the baby to breast / help the baby conserve energy.

    b. let the infant's suckling stimulate the letdown reflex / allow the infant to set the pace of the feeding.

    c. pump rapid-flow milk from the breast / ensure that the small amount of milk taken by the infant is hindmilk.

    d. pump rapid-flow milk from the breast / slow the milk flow to make breathing during nursing easier on the infant.

34. The head and neck of a small, young, less-mature preterm infant should be firmly supported at the breast for all of the following reasons *except*

    a. breastfeeding proceeds more smoothly when the infant's gaze cannot wander.

    b. infant suction pressure is lower than it will be later.

    c. the infant typically is unable to draw the nipple into his mouth.

    d. undirected head movements may collapse the infant's airway.

35. A premature infant with a weak suck may still obtain sufficient breastmilk at a feeding if all of the following are in place *except* that the

    a. infant attaches well to the breast.

    b. infant supports his own head.

    c. maternal milk supply is good.

    d. milk-ejection reflex is easily stimulated.

36. In a baby who has just been weighed before and after a breastfeeding, a 1 gram weight gain is approximately equivalent to a milk intake of _____.

    a. 0.5 ml.

    b. 0.75 ml.

    c. 1.00 ml.

    d. 1.25 ml.

37. The *best* reason for having an abundant milk supply at the time a premature infant is discharged from the hospital is that the extra milk

    a. can be frozen for future use.

    b. ensures good milk ejection when the mother nurses lying down.

    c. may compensate for a weak infant suck.

    d. will stretch the infant's stomach so he will be able to take larger volumes.

38. Use of a thin silicone nipple shield over the mother's nipple allows the infant to more easily

    a. elicit a strong milk-ejection reflex in his mother.

    b. generate suction needed to draw milk into his mouth.

    c. generate suction needed to position the breast in his mouth.

    d. obtain milk without relying on suction.

39. A mother who uses a nipple shield to encourage an immature preterm infant to feed at the breast will typically

    a. increase her infant's milk intake and her own milk yield.

    b. reduce her milk supply in the long run.

    c. reduce the amount of milk the infant is able to take.

    d. require a longer time to complete a feeding as compared with cup feeding.

40. Otherwise healthy premature infants typically are at risk of consuming too little milk at the breast until about

    a. 3 months after birth.

    b. term-corrected age.

    c. the time at which birthweight has trebled.

    d. the time that a nursing blister first forms on the infant's upper lip.

41. During the first few weeks at home, waking a premature infant more than every 3 hours is generally is _____ in order to promote adequate _____

    a. discouraged / development of state control.

    b. discouraged / release of growth hormone.

    c. encouraged / hydration.

    d. encouraged / nutrient intake.

42. Because preterm infants may have difficulty consuming sufficient milk at the breast during the first few weeks after discharge, all of the following are recommended *except* to

    a. continue use of a thin, silicone nipple shield.

    b. monitor weight gain every 2 or 3 days by test weighing on a scale accurate to 1 or 2 grams.

    c. reduce use of nipple shields beginning about 10 days after discharge home.

    d. supplement the infant with expressed breastmilk in a bottle.

Discussion Questions

1. Should a milk expression schedule for the mother of a preterm infant parallel the frequency with which a healthy, full-term newborn breastfeeds? If not, how is the schedule to be modified?

2. How can mothers who pump milk to be fed to their hospitalized infants minimize bacterial contamination of their milk? Is sterile breastmilk a realistic goal?

3. For optimal breast stimulation, should a mother pump her breasts at the same time or sequentially?

4. Which of the following best indicates that an infant is ready to feed directly from the breast?

   • The infant can suck rhythmically at his mother's soft breast.

   • The infant can take a full bottle of breastmilk.

   • The infant is no longer using supplementary oxygen.

   • The infant has reached 4 pounds in weight.

   • The infant has reached term-corrected age.

   • What is the rationale for your response?

5. Are clinical indices of milk intake at the breast adequate for assessing the intake of premature infants? What procedures ensure the validity of test weighing of infants used to determine milk intake?

6. Why are each of the following signs monitored during early breastfeeding sessions for a hospitalized premature infant?
   - Heart rate
   - Respiratory rate
   - Oxygen saturation or transcutaneous oxygen pressure (TcPO$_2$)
   - Body temperature
   - Weight before and after a feeding

7. How does the early milk of a mother who delivered a preterm infant differ from the early milk of a mother who delivered a term infant? How long will that difference persist?

8. What is the advantage to the baby of fortifying expressed mother's milk? With his own mother's hind milk? With commercial fortifiers?

9. What is skin-to-skin care (also called "kangaroo" care)? How does it benefit the infant? How does it benefit the mother?

10. What can be done to make it easier for mothers to pump their milk frequently?

11. How should expressed mother's milk be labeled and stored? At home before it is taken to the neonatal intensive care unit (NICU)? In the NICU? How should it be prepared in the NICU for feeding?

12. What is the relation between gavage infusion rates and lipid loss? Is lipid loss a problem? What is the rationale for your answer? How can lipid loss be minimized?

13. What pharmaceutical preparations may be recommended to a mother whose milk volumes are faltering? Describe guidelines for using each. Are there limits to their use?

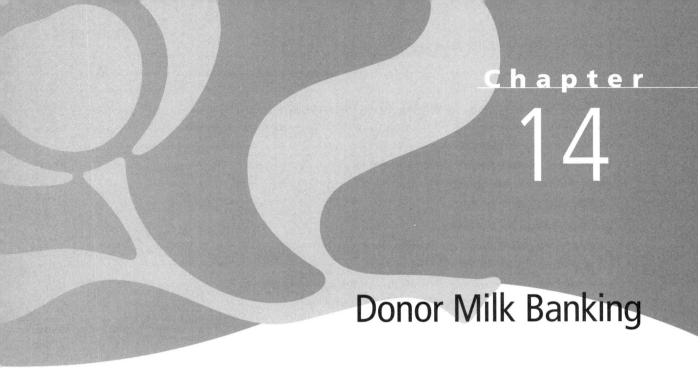

Chapter

14

Donor Milk Banking

Introduction

Banked human milk helps to bridge the gap when a mother's own milk is not available and her infant does not thrive on manufactured milks. Modern human milk banks balance a humanitarian response to those who require the nutritive or immunological properties of human milk with scrupulous practices to ensure that the banked milk will not cause infection in the recipient. Questions in this chapter will help you to assess your understanding of this body of information and how it applies to professional practice.

IBLCE Disciplines

Information in this chapter applies to the following disciplines tested on the certification examination offered by the International Board of Lactation Consultant Examiners: J = Ethical and Legal Issues; K = Breastfeeding Equipment and Technology; L = Techniques; 4 = Prematurity.

Multiple-Choice Questions

1. Banked human milk is most commonly used in which of the following situations?
   a. Infant does not tolerate artificial milks.
   b. Mother cannot take her baby with her on an extended absence from home.
   c. Mother has a healthy adopted infant.
   d. Mother is undergoing chemotherapy.

2. In addition to being used for feedings of newborn infants, banked human milk has also been used for older infants or children in all the following situations *except* when infants

    a. are healthy and adopted.

    b. are recuperating from stomach surgery.

    c. do not tolerate breastmilk substitutes.

    d. need treatment for thrush.

3. Banked human milk is least likely to benefit

    a. adults preparing for an organ transplant.

    b. children who are mending broken bones.

    c. premature infants whose own mother's milk supply failed.

    d. toddlers who are highly allergic to table foods.

4. When mother's own milk is not available, the World Health Organization and the American Academy of Pediatrics _____ the use of banked human milk _____ .

    a. discourage / because of certain cultural restrictions.

    b. discourage / because of safety issues.

    c. recommend / as the next best food.

    d. recommend / if age-appropriate formula is not available either.

5. Which milk bank procedure best insures that banked human milk is free of harmful content?

    a. Collecting milk into a sterile bottle

    b. Pasteurization of the milk

    c. Physician approval of a potential donor

    d. Screening of donor serum

6. A potential donor (2009) will be screened for antigens or antibodies to all of the following *except*

    a. hepatitis B and C.

    b. HIV 1 and 2.

    c. measles.

    d. syphilis.

7. Banked human milk can be made available to a week-old infant in response to a(n) _____ to a milk bank.

    a. order from the infant's attending physician

    b. parent's written request

    c. parent's written request plus a note confirming need from the infant's physician

    d. request from a nurse or lactation consultant helping to care for the infant

8. Lactation consultants should _____ informal sharing or purchase of breastmilk because _____ .

    a. discourage / current Canadian law and U.S. federal law regulate the sale of human milk.

    b. discourage / such milk cannot be guaranteed free of pathogens, contaminants, or diluents.

    c. encourage / it is nutritionally superior to formula.

    d. encourage / it will be fresher (more recently pumped).

9. In most countries with human milk banks, donors are not paid in order to

  a. eliminate a cost that would be passed along to the recipient's family.

  b. ensure that donors are highly motivated.

  c. reduce the number of donors to be trained.

  d. remove an incentive to sell milk needed by a donor's infant.

10. For each ounce of milk received by an infant, a fee is charged that accounts for all of the following *except*

  a. payment for the milk itself.

  b. processing the donated milk.

  c. screening donors.

  d. testing the milk for pathogens.

11. At most milk banks, all of the following temporarily disqualify a mother from donating breastmilk *except*

  a. ingestion of alcoholic drinks.

  b. tattoos or body piercings within the previous 12 months.

  c. use of medication during an acute illness.

  d. older than 35 years of age.

12. Holder pasteurization of human milk

  a. destroys bacteria but not viruses.

  b. destroys both viruses and bacteria.

  c. is not the preferred way of processing human milk at some North American milk banks.

  d. requires that milk be heated at 62.5°C for only 10 minutes.

13. Common practices among United States donor milk banks include all of the following *except*

  a. always age-matching milk and recipient by post-birth age in weeks.

  b. classifying milk as "preterm milk" for no more than 28 days after preterm birth.

  c. making milk available to babies in all 50 states.

  d. ensuring that every pool of milk is sterile before it is dispensed.

14. Milk expressed by mothers of preterm infants is pooled with milk from mothers of _____ in order to _____.

  a. other preterm infants / foster better infant growth by matching the "age" of the milk with the age of the recipient infants.

  b. other preterm infants / more easily fortify the milk before it is shipped.

  c. term infants / increase the concentration of immunologic factors in the pooled milk.

  d. term infants / increase the concentration of protein in the pooled milk.

15. Mother's own milk or banked human milk fed to preterm infants in neonatal intensive-care units has been linked in the recipient infants with all of the following *except*

  a. higher IQ at 8 years of age.

  b. less risk of necrotizing enterocolitis.

  c. lower cholesterol concentration.

  d. more days on a respirator.

Discussion Questions

1. How does the Human Milk Banking Association of North America affect the establishment or operation of a milk bank?

2. For what medical indications might banked human milk be prescribed for an infant in a neonatal intensive care unit?

3. Why do milk banks handle donor milk as few times as possible between the donor mother and the recipient infant?

4. What are conditions or practices that will cause a milk bank to decline a person as a donor? Are these conditions or practices temporary or permanent?

5. How has the fear of HIV infection affected human milk banking?

6. How is human milk processed? How is it stored?

7. How many milk banks are there in the United States at the present time? Which milk bank is closest to you? What is its approximate processing fee for banked milk?

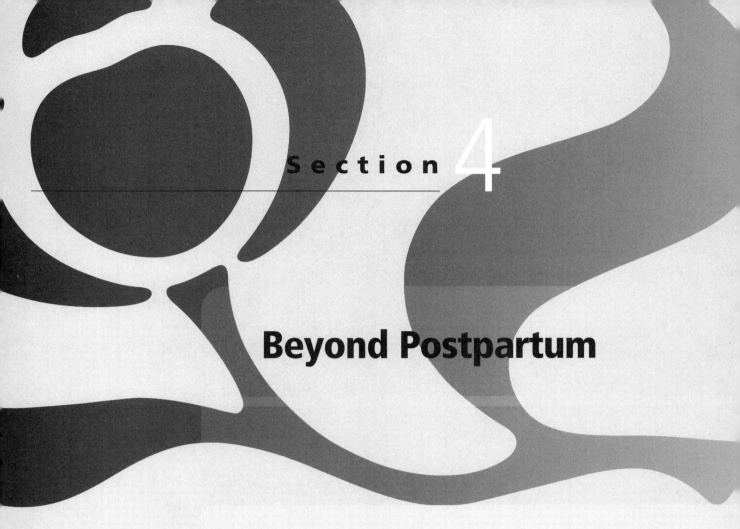

Section 4

Beyond Postpartum

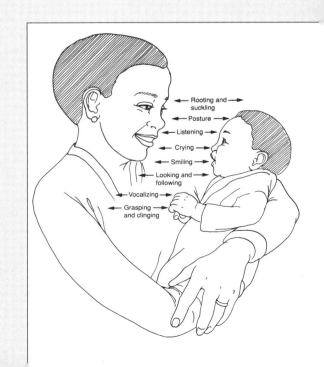

Maternal Nutrition During Lactation

Introduction

Does a mother's diet make a difference to how much breastmilk she produces? Or to her breastmilk's nutritional adequacy? Or to her baby's response to it? The answer is "Generally not—but maybe, in some circumstances." Although daily diet usually has little influence on milk composition, some dietary practices—such as strict veganism or rapid weight loss—do. Questions in this chapter will help you to assess your understanding of this body of information and how it applies to professional practice.

IBLCE Disciplines

Information in this chapter applies to the following disciplines tested on the certification examination offered by the International Board of Lactation Consultant Examiners: C = Maternal and Infant Normal Nutrition and Biochemistry; G = Psychology, Sociology, and Anthropology; 12 = General Principles.

Multiple-Choice Questions

1. The breastmilk of a chronically malnourished breastfeeding mother typically is
   a. deficient in protein.
   b. deficient in water-soluble constituents.
   c. secreted using constituents of the maternal diet.
   d. secreted using constituents of the maternal diet and body stores.

2. A malnourished breastfeeding mother typically will produce
   a. average or slightly smaller-than-average daily volumes of milk.
   b. average volumes during the first 6 weeks or so but declining volumes thereafter.
   c. milk of lower fat content.
   d. severely reduced daily volumes of milk.

3. To maintain her own body weight during exclusive breastfeeding, about how many calories in excess of her pre-pregnancy intake does a mother need?

   a. 300

   b. 500

   c. 750

   d. 900

4. About what percentage of food energy is converted to breastmilk?

   a. No more than 50

   b. 60

   c. 70

   d. At least 80

5. To remain well hydrated, a breastfeeding mother should drink

   a. at least 8 ounces per hour.

   b. only between meals.

   c. only filtered water.

   d. to quench her own thirst.

6. Forcing fluid intake beyond the need to quench maternal thirst poses the risk of

   a. diluting the milk—providing fewer calories per ounce of milk.

   b. producing more milk than the baby can use.

   c. reducing milk production.

   d. triggering edema in the breasts.

7. Early signs of dehydration in a lactating mother are constipation and

   a. dark urine.

   b. flaking skin.

   c. lack of tears.

   d. pale urine.

8. Daily food intake typically contributes about what percentage of usual water intake?

   a. 10

   b. 15

   c. 20

   d. 30

9. During the first 6 months of breastfeeding, a portion of the fat stored during pregnancy typically

   a. begins to be lost beginning with the onset of lactogenesis II.

   b. is lost even with daily ingestion of 2,600 calories.

   c. is lost gradually during the first 6 months but quite rapidly thereafter.

   d. provides about 100–150 calories per day to support milk production.

10. The maximum rate of weight loss that does not harm milk volume or composition is about _____ pound(s) per _____.

    a. 0.5 / day.

    b. 0.5 / week.

    c. 1 / week.

    d. 2 / week.

11. As compared with mothers feeding formula, in the first 6 months postpartum breastfeeding mothers tend to lose

    a. about the same amount of weight.

    b. less weight because they have a greater food intake.

    c. more weight because they are more active.

    d. more weight despite being less active.

12. Extremely rapid maternal weight loss by a breastfeeding woman may cause

    a. environmental toxins to move in larger quantities from fat stores into breastmilk.

    b. extreme placidity in the infant as fat shifts into the milk.

    c. increased rate of infant weight gain as fat shifts into the milk.

    d. opening of leaky junctions between lactocytes.

13. Moderate (not to exhaustion) exercise by lactating women has been shown to _____ of breastmilk.

    a. decrease the daily total milk volume

    b. decrease the lactose content

    c. increase the daily total milk volume

    d. increase the lactic acid content

14. Women who breastfeed following gastric bypass surgery to correct morbid obesity _____ breast-feed because _____

    a. may, if supervised by a physician, / a wide range of maternal nutrient absorption can allow normal compositions of milk.

    b. may / the surgery only minimally reduces absorption of nutrients.

    c. should not / there is a high risk of synthesizing milk lacking minerals.

    d. should not / there is a high risk of synthesizing milk low in fats.

15. A healthy mother who increases her calcium intake while breastfeeding

    a. may reduce absorption of iron and magnesium.

    b. reduces her risk of osteoporosis later in life.

    c. tends to increase the calcium concentration in her breastmilk.

    d. will prevent the slight bone loss that is common during lactation.

16. The risk of later hip fracture in women who breastfed one or more children

    a. decreases in women who supplement dietary calcium and phosphorus.

    b. increases in women who breastfeed more than 6 months.

    c. increases with each child breastfed.

    d. is inversely related to the total duration of breastfeeding.

17. Reduction of bone density during lactation is all of the following *except*
    a. associated with early resumption of menses.
    b. compensated for after weaning.
    c. more severe with each subsequent child breastfed.
    d. temporary.

18. Women who consume lacto-ovo vegetarian diets produce breastmilk that
    a. generally is nutritionally adequate.
    b. generally is not nutritionally adequate.
    c. may be low in calcium and vitamin B_{12}.
    d. may be low in energy content.

19. As of 2009, the Women, Infants, and Children Program of the U.S. Department of Health and Human Services provides food supplements to qualifying lactating mothers for ____ months.
    a. 3
    b. 6
    c. 8
    d. 12

20. Rickets in breastfed infants can be avoided by
    a. breastfeeding as usual.
    b. increasing calcium intake in the mother.
    c. supplementing the infant with vitamin D.
    d. supplementing the mother with vitamin D.

21. A very young breastfeeding infant whose mother ingests moderate amounts of caffeine is likely to
    a. break down caffeine in his small intestine.
    b. ingest caffeine that passed into breastmilk, but in a very low dose.
    c. sleep less, if he is full term and healthy.
    d. sleep more if he is premature because he metabolizes caffeine only poorly.

22. Foods ingested by a lactating mother
    a. are the cause of most nursing "strikes."
    b. can expose the infant to medicinal concentrations of some compounds.
    c. prepare an infant to more easily accept family table foods.
    d. rarely impart any flavor to breastmilk.

23. Which of the following statements is false? A mother's tissue concentration of the heavy metal(s)
    a. lead and mercury is more harmful to the infant during pregnancy than during lactation.
    b. lead is increased by high maternal concentrations of calcium and phosphorus.
    c. mercury can be reduced by avoiding excessive consumption of fish or of cow milk from animals fed fish products.
    d. mercury is not increased by the mercury in dental fillings sufficiently to harm the infant through breastmilk.

24. The *most* common food ingested by a lactating woman that produces an allergic response in her infant is
    a. citrus fruit.
    b. dairy products.
    c. peanuts.
    d. wheat.

25. Mothers in all of the following categories *except* one are at nutritional risk during lactation. Which one?
    a. Age 35 or over
    b. Maternal weight less than 85 percent of optimal weight
    c. Rapid weight loss while breastfeeding
    d. Small weight gain during pregnancy

26. The component of breastmilk that most closely reflects maternal dietary intake is
    a. calcium.
    b. carbohydrates.
    c. lipids.
    d. protein.

27. The energy density of fat is about _____ that of carbohydrate or of protein.
    a. half
    b. 10 percent more than
    c. the same as
    d. twice

28. The vitamin content of breastmilk is more likely to reflect _____ if the vitamins are _____.
    a. maternal body stores / B or C.
    b. maternal body stores / water soluble.
    c. recent dietary intake / A, D, E, or K.
    d. recent dietary intake / water soluble.

29. A lactating woman who intends to consume alcohol should _____ special precautions and _____.
    a. take / consume food along with only small amounts of alcoholic drinks.
    b. take / ingest alcohol on an empty stomach to get it out of her system more rapidly.
    c. take no / because it will be rendered harmless in the infant's stomach.
    d. take no / because little alcohol passes into breastmilk.

30. As compared with the iron ingested by formula-fed infants, the iron ingested by breastfed infants is
    a. less efficiently metabolized.
    b. metabolized at about the same efficiency as iron in formula.
    c. more efficiently metabolized, but the low iron content of breastmilk puts the infant at risk of anemia.
    d. such that the breastfed infant is at less risk of anemia.

Discussion   Questions

1. How many extra calories, on average, does a woman need to support adequate breastmilk production? Why is that number so small?

2. What would you advise a mother who wishes to begin a weight loss program when her baby is 4 weeks old?

3. What is the relation between intensity of maternal exercise and infant refusal to breastfeed? Does this mean lactating women can't exercise at all? What is the rationale for your answer?

4. What are the main kinds of vegetarian diets? Do any of them compromise the health of a breastfeeding infant? If so, in what way? How can any deficiency be corrected?

5. What is the effect of a woman drinking several (say, five) cups of coffee a day on her breastfeeding infant? Does the woman need to cut down or cut out her coffee consumption? Does the same hold true if the infant is premature?

6. What are micronutrients? Name three and describe the effect on an infant of a deficiency in each.

7. Does breastfeeding contribute to osteoporosis in the mother? During lactation? Later in life? What is the rationale for your response?

8. Are vitamin supplements necessary for a breastfeeding mother?

9. Does maternal ingestion of highly flavored foods irritate her breastfeeding infant? Should a lactating woman's own diet be bland? What is the rationale for your response?

10. Do teenage breastfeeding mothers require different nutritional guidelines than older breastfeeding mothers? What is the rationale for your response?

11. A mother asks you if it is all right to drink wine at an upcoming party. How do answers to the following questions influence your advice?
    - How far along in her pregnancy is the mother?
    - How many ounces of wine might the mother drink?
    - Will food also be served?

Women's Health and Breastfeeding

Introduction

When a breastfeeding mother is ill—whether the illness is acute or chronic—several questions must be answered: How does the illness affect breastfeeding? How does breastfeeding affect the illness? What will be the physiological and the psychological effects if the baby is weaned in response to his mother's illness? If breastfeeding continues, how can the baby be nourished and protected in the face of his mother's illness? Questions in this chapter will help you to assess your understanding of this body of information and how it applies to professional practice

IBLCE Disciplines

Information in this chapter applies to the following disciplines tested on the certification examination offered by the International Board of Lactation Consultant Examiners: C = Maternal and Infant Normal Nutrition and Biochemistry; D = Maternal and Infant Immunology and Infectious Disease; E = Maternal and Infant Pathology; F = Maternal and Infant Pharmacology and Toxicology.

Multiple-Choice Questions

1. For each additional year that a woman lactates, she has a _____ percent decrease in the risk of diabetes later in life.

   a. 5

   b. 15

   c. 25

   d. 40

2. Women in whom gestational diabetes develops during pregnancy are *best* advised to _____, because _____.

    a. breastfeed / it reduces the risk of developing type II diabetes later on.

    b. breastfeed / they will lose weight more rapidly postpartum.

    c. not breastfeed / of increased risk of mastitis.

    d. not breastfeed / lactation impairs maternal glucose metabolism.

3. As compared with healthy nondiabetic women, women with type I diabetes experience lactogenesis II about a day _____, typically because _____.

    a. earlier / blood glucose concentrations are higher.

    b. earlier / thyroid concentrations are higher.

    c. later / blood glucose concentrations are lower.

    d. later / prolactin concentrations are lower.

4. After parturition, a mother with type I diabetes will excrete _____ in her urine.

    a. glucose

    b. fructose

    c. lactose

    d. sucrose

5. As compared with diabetic mothers who do not breastfeed, diabetic mothers who do breastfeed have blood glucose concentrations that generally average

    a. about the same, assuming that each set of mothers adjusts caloric intake to keep blood glucose within proper limits.

    b. markedly lower, despite the higher caloric intake of breastfeeding mothers.

    c. somewhat higher, because of the higher caloric intake of breastfeeding mothers.

    d. very slightly lower, in women who correctly balance additional calories with infant withdrawal of milk.

6. The injected insulin taken by breastfeeding women with type I diabetes _____ pass to the infant in breastmilk, _____.

    a. does / but in such small quantities that the infant adjusts his milk intake to account for it.

    b. does / but is destroyed in the infant's gastrointestinal system.

    c. does not / because insulin has little protein-binding capacity.

    d. does not / because the insulin molecule is too large to pass into lactocytes.

7. Women with diabetes who breastfeed

    a. may be at greater risk of mastitis than are other breastfeeding women.

    b. may be at less risk for candidiasis than are other breastfeeding women.

    c. should withhold colostrum until their own blood glucose has stabilized.

    d. will likely need more insulin than they did during pregnancy.

8. Candidiasis in a breastfeeding diabetic mother is promoted by all of the following *except*

    a. elevated blood glucose concentration.

    b. lowered blood glucose concentration.

    c. a nipple that remains damp after a feeding.

    d. other concurrent infection.

9. A diabetic mother who is ready to wean her infant should wean _____, because she can then _____.
   a. rapidly / adjust her own metabolism more quickly.
   b. rapidly / enjoy an interval of high calorie intake.
   c. slowly / gradually decrease her food intake.
   d. slowly / gradually decrease her insulin dosage.

10. A mother who presents with low milk supply, poor infant growth, constantly feeling chilled, and thin hair may have diminished _____ secretion.
    a. cortisol
    b. dopamine
    c. prolactin
    d. thyroid

11. Severe postpartum hemorrhage can result in injury to the _____ that leads to _____.
    a. hypothalamus / lactation failure.
    b. hypothalamus / prolactin-secreting tumors and galactorrhea.
    c. pituitary / lactation failure.
    d. pituitary / prolactin-secreting tumors and galactorrhea.

12. Mothers with cystic fibrosis generally _____ be encouraged to breastfeed, because _____.
    a. should / breastfeeding will help to maintain maternal weight.
    b. should / the milk is nourishing and will protect the infant from maternal pathogens.
    c. should not / of the high concentration of maternal bacterial pathogens.
    d. should not / the fat profile of the breastmilk is abnormal.

13. A mother with cystic fibrosis can continue breastfeeding as long as she
    a. loses weight slowly.
    b. remains in stable health.
    c. takes vitamin D supplements.
    d. supplements her infant with formula.

14. A breastfeeding mother who contracts an acute illness, such as influenza, should _____ wean in order to _____.
    a. not / pass along antibodies to her illness to her infant.
    b. not / pass along the therapeutic dose of her medication to her infant.
    c. temporarily / avoid exposing her infant to her illness.
    d. temporarily / avoid exposing her infant to medications used to combat the illness.

15. During her treatment, a mother with tuberculosis
    a. cannot breastfeed because her milk volumes will be very small.
    b. should interrupt breastfeeding temporarily at the outset of treatment.
    c. should not breastfeed at all to avoid infecting her infant through her milk.
    d. should not breastfeed at all to avoid contact infection of her infant.

16. Methicillin-resistant *Staphylococcus aureus* (MRSA) infection in neonates immediately after birth can be reduced by all of the following *except*
    a. allowing any medical staff free access to the infant.
    b. ample skin-to-skin contact.
    c. holding and nursing the baby in the delivery room.
    d. keeping the baby physically close during rooming in.

17. Excessive postpartum uterine bleeding may be related to
    a. abundant milk supply.
    b. fragments of placenta retained in the uterus.
    c. gestational diabetes.
    d. low infant Apgar scores.

18. Putting a neonate to breast in the early postpartum can reduce maternal blood loss because suckling
    a. causes uterine contractions.
    b. decreases the diameter of small blood vessels.
    c. increases the viscosity of the blood.
    d. stimulates the production of clotting factors.

19. Standard immunizations using vaccines that contain killed or attenuated micro-organisms generally are *best* offered to a breastfeeding woman
    a. after complete weaning to ensure an active immune response.
    b. after her infant has begun a secondary food source.
    c. as needed by the woman irrespective of breastfeeding status.
    d. before complete weaning so that the infant can receive a secondary dose.

20. A breastfeeding mother who must be hospitalized for surgery should be encouraged to do all of the following *except*
    a. arrange to have her infant room in with her.
    b. breastfeed as late before and as soon after surgery as possible.
    c. learn about hospital services for lactating women.
    d. wean the baby in advance of surgery.

21. The American Red Cross recommends that lactating women wait at least _____ weeks after an uncomplicated term delivery before donating blood.
    a. 6
    b. 12
    c. 26
    d. 52

22. Research supports that inducing milk production after an untimely weaning from the breast is easier if all of the following are true *except* that the
    a. baby accepts the breast willingly.
    b. baby is less than about 3 months old.
    c. interval between the baby's birth and the untimely weaning is short.
    d. mother uses blessed thistle or fenugreek seed infusions to increase her milk supply.

23. The hormonal milieu required for synthesis of breastmilk requires
    a. a functional uterus.
    b. a preceding pregnancy, even if interrupted.
    c. functional ovaries.
    d. nipple stimulation.

24. Domperidone and metoclopramide are commonly used
    a. analgesics.
    b. galactogogues.
    c. milk suppressants.
    d. tranquilizers.

25. The volume of milk synthesized by an adoptive mother without a previous pregnancy depends *primarily* on
    a. how long she is able to pump her breasts before the baby arrives.
    b. the degree of the mother's motivation.
    c. the vigor with which the infant suckles.
    d. whether the mother has functioning ovaries.

26. An infant being reestablished at the breast after an interval of formula feedings will pass stools that have a(n)
    a. firmer consistency.
    b. increasingly unpleasant odor.
    c. larger volume.
    d. paler, more yellow color.

27. Breastfeeding by a woman who has multiple sclerosis, a progressive degenerative neurologic disorder, should be _____, because _____.
    a. discouraged / of the physical demands on the mother's body.
    b. discouraged / the medications commonly prescribed are considered risky for the infant.
    c. encouraged / a factor in her milk may protect the infant from later developing the disease.
    d. encouraged / it extends the remission of symptoms experienced during pregnancy.

28. Symptoms of rheumatoid arthritis, a chronic inflammatory disease thought to be caused by an autoimmune response, typically
    a. are less apt to develop in women who lactate for at least 2 years.
    b. decrease during lactation, because of higher concentrations of prolactin.
    c. go into remission during pregnancy and the postpartum interval.
    d. increase during lactation, stimulated by higher concentrations of dopamine.

29. Injury to the spinal cord affects lactation in all of the following ways *except*
    a. below the 1st thoracic vertebra the mother can position her infant at the breast.
    b. below the 6th cervical vertebra it is probable that the mother can lactate.
    c. between the 4th and 6th thoracic vertebra the milk ejection reflex is diminished.
    d. between the 4th and 6th thoracic vertebra thyroid secretion is diminished.

30. A breastfeeding mother with epilepsy
    a. can breastfeed if her infant is monitored for drug reactions.
    b. is more likely to drop her infant than is an epileptic mother who bottle feeds.
    c. must forgo her treatment regimen during the course of breastfeeding.
    d. should not consider breastfeeding.

31. Migraine headaches
    a. delay their postpartum recurrence in a breastfeeding mother.
    b. increase in intensity throughout a pregnancy.
    c. may be linked to the suckling-induced elevation of prolactin.
    d. treated with standard drugs require a 6-hour interval during which the baby does not nurse.

32. A mother who experiences postpartum depression is *most* likely to
    a. be especially sensitive to postpartum hormonal changes.
    b. be in her mid-30s or older.
    c. have a stressful life with little emotional support.
    d. have had a high-risk pregnancy.

33. Major postpartum depression
    a. can be alleviated by Saint-John's-wort.
    b. has little effect on the young infant if other people in the household are loving.
    c. is typically treated with medications that the infant eliminates poorly.
    d. may disrupt the formation of the bond between mother and infant.

34. A mother using medications to control her asthma and who wishes to breastfeed generally should be _____ because _____.
    a. discouraged / her medications pose a risk to the infant.
    b. discouraged / oxytocin surges narrow air passages in the lungs.
    c. encouraged / breastfeeding may help protect her infant from asthma.
    d. encouraged / oxytocin surges cause air passages to expand.

35. Maternal cigarette smoking during the course of breastfeeding decreases the
    a. carbon monoxide levels in the infant.
    b. fat content in her breastmilk.
    c. risk of maternal breast abscess.
    d. risk of respiratory illness in the infant.

36. If his mother smokes cigarettes daily, an infant is better off being fed
    a. at the breast, because nicotine is inert in the infant's system.
    b. at the breast, to obtain the nutritional and immunological benefits of breastmilk.
    c. formula, to avoid ingesting nicotine-containing breastmilk.
    d. formula, to minimize handling by a mother who carries an aura of cigarette smoke.

37. A mother who develops contact dermatitis from poison ivy _____ breastfeeding _____.

    a. can continue / if she is comfortable enough to do so.

    b. should continue / to pass resistance to poison ivy dermatitis to her infant through her milk.

    c. should discontinue / because breastfeeding will only exacerbate her discomfort.

    d. should discontinue / so that the infant will not risk acquiring poison ivy dermatitis from the mother's skin eruptions.

Discussion Questions

1. What is the difference between an acute and a chronic illness? Describe an example of each.

2. What are at least four ways in which a lactating woman can prepare to minimize separation or interruption of breastfeeding caused by her own surgery? Her infant's surgery?

3. How does cigarette smoking affect women, as a group, in their breastfeeding course?

4. What is a prolactinoma? What restrictions does it place on breastfeeding?

5. During a lactating woman's self-limiting acute illness, should she as a general rule interrupt breastfeeding? By continuing to breastfeed, does the infant obtain any benefits? Does the infant incur any risk?

6. Do any maternal illnesses preclude breastfeeding? Is the illness the problem, or the treatment for the illness?

7. Severe postpartum hemorrhage in a new mother may be associated with what breastfeeding outcome? Describe the physiology causing this outcome.

8. What physiological pathways allow induced lactation (as in the case of an adopted infant) to succeed to some degree? Why then do most adoptive mothers who induce lactation also offer supplements to their infants? Discuss at least two factors in the mother and two in the infant that may make it difficult for the mother to bring in a full milk supply.

9. How can a physically impaired mother, a mother with a seizure disorder, or a mother with rheumatoid arthritis manage breastfeeding? Is breastfeeding inherently riskier to the baby's safety than formula feeding? How do you justify your answer?

10. What is the difference between relactation and induced lactation? What are the potential benefits of each? Are there any potential risks or other downsides?

11. What are three degrees of postpartum depression? Are they affected by the normal postpartum shifts in hormones? Does breastfeeding influence the course of postpartum depression?

12. Does a woman who smokes face any increased health risks related to breastfeeding? Does her infant face any health risks related to his mother's cigarette smoking?

13. Can breastfeeding and headache be related? What physiology underlies the connection? What are some suggestions to help the mother cope?

Maternal Employment and Breastfeeding

Introduction

Maintaining breastfeeding while being employed outside the home isn't particularly easy, but in many circumstances it is possible. A lactation consultant can advise on accommodations concerning the workplace, family life (especially sleeping), day care, and pumping that facilitate continued breastfeeding. Questions in this chapter will help you to assess your understanding of this body of information and how it applies to professional practice.

IBLCE Disciplines

Information in this chapter applies to the following disciplines tested on the certification examination offered by the International Board of Lactation Consultant Examiners: G = Psychology, Sociology, and Anthropology; K = Breastfeeding Equipment and Technology; L = Techniques; M = Public Health.

Multiple-Choice Questions

1. A working mother is more likely to breastfeed for a longer total duration if all the following are true *except*

   a. her infant is older when she returns to work.

   b. she combines breastfeeding with formula feeding.

   c. she feeds breastmilk exclusively after her return to work.

   d. she works part time rather than full time.

2. Mothers employed outside the home who view breastfeeding as a special time with her infant are inclined to

   a. breastfeed a shorter time after returning to work, because of difficulty in maintaining earlier routines.

   b. breastfeed longer only if employed 20 hours per week or less.

   c. breastfeed longer, even if they are employed full time.

   d. completely wean upon returning to work and set new routines in place with her infant.

3. The *most* common reason offered by employed women who wean early is

   a. insufficient milk supply.

   b. lack of knowledge about managing breastfeeding in the workplace.

   c. lack of time to pump.

   d. unsupportive workplace.

4. Factors promoting continuation of breastfeeding by employed mothers include all of the following *except*

   a. brief maternity leave, so that little catch-up is required when she returns to work.

   b. flexible work schedule, so she can feed or pump as needed.

   c. on-site child care, so she can breastfeed her infant during the day.

   d. supportive workplace, so she is among people who appreciate her effort.

5. A mother will be better prepared to continue breastfeeding after returning to work if she has learned how to do all of the following *except*

   a. maintain her milk supply.

   b. store breastmilk.

   c. train her infant to take a bottle.

   d. use various types of breast pump.

6. As compared with women who are employed full time, women who work part time breastfeed for

   a. a longer duration.

   b. a shorter duration.

   c. about the same duration, but they introduce complementary foods later.

   d. about the same duration, but they introduce complementary foods earlier.

7. Infants placed in group child care have an increased incidence of

   a. *Candida* (thrush) infections.

   b. diarrhea.

   c. infections related to teething.

   d. lower respiratory infection.

8. As compared with breastfeeding mothers who do not express milk at work, mothers who do express breastmilk while they are at work are _____ likely to _____.

   a. less / have good relationships with their coworkers.

   b. less / miss work because of illness in her infant.

   c. more / miss work because of plugged ducts or mastitis.

   d. more / reduce their milk supply.

9. In the United States, Transportation Security Administration rules allow human milk to be carried on board an airplane in bottles that
   a. cannot be opened without breaking a seal applied to the cap.
   b. hold less than 3 ounces.
   c. may contain more than 3 ounces.
   d. Only a and c.

10. The bacterial concentration in expressed human milk
    a. falls during the first few hours after expression only if it is immediately refrigerated.
    b. falls during the first few hours after expression even if it remains at room temperature.
    c. rises gradually beginning about an hour after the milk was expressed, if it remains at room temperature.
    d. rises sharply beginning about an hour after the milk was expressed, if it remains at room temperature.

11. Refrigeration of expressed milk for as much as 8 days, as compared with _____, is recommended to better retain _____.
    a. immediate freezing / antimicrobial factors.
    b. immediate freezing / fats.
    c. immediate freezing / sodium-transport proteins.
    d. longer refrigeration / vitamin C.

12. Milk that is frozen at home (in a refrigerator freezer with a separate door)
    a. best nourishes the baby if milk is used as soon as possible.
    b. may be used up to 6 months later.
    c. should be placed near the door, to allow more rapid access to stored milk.
    d. that was warmed for a bottle feeding, but remained in the bottle at the end of the feeding, may be stored for 48 hours.

13. A portion of thawed breastmilk that remains after a bottle feeding
    a. may be layered on top of still-frozen milk and refrozen.
    b. may be left at room temperature if the next feeding will be within 3 hours.
    c. should be discarded.
    d. should be promptly refrigerated and used at the next feeding.

14. Expressed breastmilk stored in a workplace break-room refrigerator
    a. may be touched or moved only by the mother who stored it.
    b. requires no special handling or storage precautions.
    c. requires special storage away from other food items that might contaminate the milk.
    d. requires special storage away from other food items that might be contaminated by the milk.

15. When freshly pumped milk is added to already frozen milk, the container should be labeled with the date on which the
    a. oldest (lowest) milk was pumped.
    b. oldest milk should no longer be used.
    c. milk is estimated to be used.
    d. youngest (highest) milk was pumped.

16. To prepare chilled or frozen milk for a feeding
    a. handle carefully to maintain the cream portion separate.
    b. heat by running warm water over the container of milk.
    c. heat in a microwave oven to body temperature.
    d. warm to room temperature on a counter.

17. "Reverse-cycle" nursing refers to
    a. a pattern of feeding more at night than during the day.
    b. an electric breast pump's adjustment of the vacuum-and-release cycle.
    c. breastfeeding on the weekend in the same pattern used during the work week.
    d. breastfeeding on the weekend just to the point of comfort, to avoid the need to express additional milk at work early the following week.

18. Women who work for companies that support continued breastfeeding among their employees by use of formal programs tend to do all of the following *except*
    a. breastfeed for longer durations, at least 6 months.
    b. feel lowered morale as an employee.
    c. make less use of company healthcare insurance for infant illness.
    d. miss fewer days of work.

19. Breastfeeding outside the home is protected or promoted in the United States by all of the following *except*
    a. a federal act that permits a mother to breastfeed anywhere that she is authorized to be.
    b. a federal act that permits breastfeeding on federal property any place that the mother is authorized to be.
    c. some state laws that remove breastfeeding in public from the category of "indecent exposure."
    d. some state laws that require employers to accommodate the pumping needs of breastfeeding employees.

20. All of the following characterize a mother who wishes to maintain her milk supply after returning to full-time employment, *except* one. She will pump
    a. at least twice during a 10-hour absence from her infant.
    b. for a total daily time, on average, of about 90 minutes.
    c. less frequently for an older baby (3–6 months of age).
    d. more frequently for a younger baby (less than 3 months of age).

Discussion Questions

1. Considering the time and effort required to pump breastmilk for their infant, why do mothers continue to do so? What are the advantages to the infant? What are advantages to the employed mother? What are advantages to her employer? What disadvantages may affect the employer?

2. What conditions allow a mother to comfortably breastfeed or pump at her work site?

3. What factors should a mother consider as she arranges day care for her infant? What should the day care provider know about breastfeeding infants? How will milk be offered to the infant? Can the mother tell if the baby has been given manufactured milk feedings without the mother's approval? How?

4. What illnesses are common in infants placed in day care? What effect does breastfeeding have on the likelihood that the breastfed infant will fall ill?

5. Whose support does a breastfeeding mother need in order to continue breastfeeding after returning to work? What do these people do to support continued breastfeeding?

6. Is a longer pumping session necessarily a "better" pumping session, if volume of milk obtained is the criterion? What combination of pumping frequency and duration maximizes the amount of milk that can be pumped in a day?

7. When is an employed mother likely to experience each of the following? How can she minimize each?
   • Engorgement or leaking
   • The baby's frequent changes of feeding patterns
   • Concern about an inadequate or fluctuating milk supply
   • The need to express or pump milk

8. What considerations control when a breastfeeding mother returns to paid employment? If the mother has some flexibility, how might she phase back in to her employment?

9. Sponsoring a program that supports breastfeeding employees requires a major commitment from employers.
   • What concerns might an employer have about a workplace lactation-support program?
   • How might those concerns be addressed? What benefits might accrue to an employer who adopts such a program?

10. What job options, other than full-time (40 hours per week) employment might be available to breastfeeding mothers who are looking for work?

11. Consider women working in typically low-paying jobs such as waitress, sales clerk, fast-food worker, child-care worker, parking-lot attendant, hotel maid, farm labor.
   • What barriers to maintaining breastfeeding after return to work are these women likely to face?
   • What coping strategies can you suggest?

Child Health

Introduction

How does breastfeeding affect the normal development and health of young children? How do feeding behaviors change as an infant grows? Questions in this chapter will help you to assess your understanding of
this body of information and how it applies to professional practice.

IBLCE Disciplines

Information in this chapter applies to the following disciplines tested on the certification examination of-
fered by the International Board of Lactation Consultant Examiners: C = Maternal and Infant Normal
Nutrition and Biochemistry; H = Growth Parameters and Developmental Milestones; I = Interpretation of
Research; 5 = 0–2 days; 10 = 7–12 months; 11 = Beyond 12 months; 12 = General Principles.

Multiple-Choice Questions

1. Studies have shown that, as compared with infants fed manufactured milk, infants fed human milk—
   even by bottle and in the absence of maternal contact—score _____ on I.Q. tests.
   a. about the same
   b. higher
   c. higher in developing countries but about the same in industrialized ones.
   d. lower

2. Motor development in a child progresses from
   a. control of large muscles to control of small ones.
   b. control of small muscles to control of large ones.
   c. feet and legs to arms and neck.
   d. trunk first, then legs, then arms.

3. As compared with his birth weight and length, at 12 months of age a baby usually has
   a. doubled both weight and length.
   b. doubled weight and increased length by half.
   c. tripled weight and doubled length.
   d. tripled weight and increased length by half.

4. As compared with formula-fed infants, after about 4 months of age breastfed infants weigh slightly
   a. less because they have less body fat.
   b. less but have more body fat.
   c. less in the United States but not elsewhere in the world.
   d. more but have less body fat.

5. In a malnourished infant, _____ is the last index of growth to be reduced.
   a. circumference of chest
   b. head circumference
   c. length from head to foot
   d. length of torso

6. Which of the following senses are well developed in full-term neonates?
   a. Hearing, taste, smell
   b. Sight, hearing, smell
   c. Smell, sight, hearing
   d. Taste, smell, sight

7. _____ infants recognize axillary odors of their mother.
   a. Both breastfed and formula-fed
   b. Neither breastfed nor formula-fed
   c. Only breastfed
   d. Only formula-fed

8. Neonates tend to be calmed by sounds that are all of the following *except*
   a. familiar as compared with unfamiliar voices.
   b. higher pitch.
   c. lower pitch.
   d. soft volume.

9. Neonates generally prefer to look at objects that share all of the following characteristics *except*
   a. about 10 inches from their eyes.
   b. in motion.
   c. monochromatic.
   d. resemble a face.

10. An infant who _____ possesses a fully developed central nervous system.

    a. blinks his eyes when relaxed

    b. coordinates suck, swallow, and gag reflex

    c. has a strong startle reflex

    d. moves steadily between alert, fussy, and sleep states

11. The young infant can *best* react to or investigate his environment when he is in a(n) _____ state, because _____

    a. alert, inactive / he can be receptive to stimuli presented to him.

    b. drowsy / he does not become overstimulated.

    c. fussy / mild internal discomfort drives efforts to control his environment.

    d. quiet, awake / he can follow visual targets or sounds.

12. As compared with infants fed formula, breastfed infants usually sleep

    a. later into the morning.

    b. longer intervals during the day.

    c. more in the late afternoon and early evening.

    d. shorter intervals during night and day.

13. With respect to social interactions, neonates are _____ and respond _____.

    a. active / but in an unfocused way to caregiver cues.

    b. active / by initiating actions to elicit a desired response from the caregiver.

    c. passive / only to their own internal needs.

    d. passive / only to their own internal needs and to strong caregiver cues.

14. A study by Harlow and Harlow (1965) demonstrated that monkey infants—and likely also human infants—perceive their mother (or other principal caregiver) principally as a source of

    a. companionship.

    b. food that relieves hunger.

    c. guidance in developing adult traits.

    d. reassurance through soft physical contact.

15. In the first hour or so after an uncomplicated and unmedicated birth, a neonate is most apt to be

    a. alert and seeking interaction with his mother.

    b. drowsy and seeking a comfortable position in which to doze.

    c. fussy or upset as he transitions into his new world.

    d. passive but receptive to attempts of parents to interact with him.

16. The end of a particular feeding is more apt to be decided by the

    a. infant, if the baby is breastfed.

    b. infant, if the baby is bottle fed.

    c. mother and baby jointly, if the infant is breastfed.

    d. mother, if the baby is breastfed.

17. Skin-to-skin (kangaroo) care of ill newborns benefits the infant *principally* because it helps to
    a. bond the mother and infant to each other.
    b. increase his mother's milk supply.
    c. keep the infant's body temperature stable.
    d. keep the infant's nares colonized with his mother's benign skin bacteria.

18. When an injection is to be given to an infant or toddler, the child's crying can be reduced if the mother does all of the following *except* _____ the child.
    a. breastfeed
    b. hold
    c. maintain skin-to-skin contact with
    d. smile at

19. Early neonatal exposure to rubella virus in breastmilk _____ in the infant.
    a. diminishes the response to later rubella vaccination
    b. does not alter the response to later rubella vaccination
    c. increases the risk of rubella developing
    d. strengthens the response to later rubella vaccination

20. As compared with the immunization of infants fed formula, the immunization of breastfeeding infants
    a. may result in higher antibody concentrations.
    b. should be avoided in order to avoid an adverse reaction to the immunization medium.
    c. should be delayed until after weaning to ensure that the immunization "takes."
    d. should be on a different schedule.

21. Vitamin D deficiency in an infant is promoted by all of the following *except*
    a. little exposure of infant skin to sunshine.
    b. low infant vitamin C stores at birth.
    c. low maternal stores of vitamin D during pregnancy.
    d. normal vitamin D content of breastmilk.

22. The American Academy of Pediatrics does not routinely recommend vitamin supplements for breast-fed infants with the exception of vitamin
    a. A.
    b. C.
    c. D.
    d. E.

23. As compared with bottle-fed older infants, breastfed older infants have _____ dental caries, in part because _____.
    a. fewer / breastmilk contains a markedly lower concentration of sugar.
    b. fewer / during a breastfeeding, nipple pores rest near the soft palate.
    c. more / lactose breaks down to sucrose, which promotes dental caries.
    d. more / they feed more frequently than bottle-fed infants.

24. As compared with bottle-fed infants, breastfed infants have a lower incidence of all of the following *except*

    a. malocclusion.

    b. thumb sucking.

    c. nasal breathing.

    d. tongue thrusting.

25. The tongue-extrusion reflex, which aids breastfeeding but hinders spoon feeding, diminishes around age _____ months.

    a. 2

    b. 4

    c. 6

    d. 8

26. Offering soft solids, such as cereals, to infants at bedtime generally will

    a. increase the time it takes the infant to fall asleep, but not change the frequency of night waking.

    b. decrease the time required to fall asleep but increase night waking.

    c. increase the time it takes to fall asleep but reduce night waking.

    d. produce no change in the infant's usual sleep pattern.

27. When soft solids are added gradually to an infant's diet, the average total daily caloric intake _____ for _____ infants.

    a. increases / breastfed.

    b. decreases / breastfed.

    c. decreases / formula-fed.

    d. remains about the same / breastfed.

28. After solids are added to an infant's diet, he will _____ water in addition, because _____.

    a. need / solid foods produce a higher osmolar load in the infant.

    b. need / to rinse any solid food clinging to the inside of his mouth, so he gets a full serving.

    c. not need / breastmilk or formula contain all the water that the infant needs.

    d. not need / solid foods contain considerable water.

29. Foods whose introduction should be delayed until well past 6 months include all of the following *except*

    a. cow milk.

    b. egg white.

    c. honey.

    d. rice.

30. Solids added to an infant's diet are *best* offered

    a. in as close to their natural state as possible.

    b. salted, to keep him from overeating.

    c. sugared, to gain easier acceptance.

    d. well cooked, to promote easy digestion.

31. Foods most likely to be accepted when added to a breastfed infant's diet include all of the following *except*

    a. cereal moistened with breastmilk.

    b. foods consumed by his mother during the course of breastfeeding.

    c. foods consumed by his mother during pregnancy.

    d. foods to which his mother is allergic.

32. If the solids added to an infant's diet are principally starches, continued breastfeeding beyond 1 year of age typically

    a. decreases the rate of infant's weight gain.

    b. depletes maternal body stores excessively.

    c. increases the likelihood of dental caries.

    d. increases the rate of linear growth in the toddler.

33. Infants fed a vegan diet may need supplements of all of the following *except*

    a. iron

    b. vitamin B_{12}.

    c. vitamin C.

    d. zinc.

34. The World Health Organization and public health organizations in the United States recommend breastfeeding

    a. no longer than through the baby's second year.

    b. through at least the baby's first year.

    c. until the baby has erupted both upper and lower incisors.

    d. until the baby has trebled his birth weight.

35. Benefits of delaying introduction of solids until around 6 months include all of the following *except*

    a. enough infant enzyme to metabolize fats.

    b. enough infant enzyme to metabolize starches.

    c. sufficient infant IgA to prevent absorption of food antigens through the intestinal wall.

    d. wide latitude on the order in which foods are introduced to the infant.

36. As compared with formula-fed infants, breastfed infants of obese parents are _____ likely to become obese themselves, because _____.

    a. less / a factor in breastmilk alters the genes responsible for a tendency to obesity.

    b. less / breastfed infants regulate their own intake.

    c. more / breastfed infants have a higher protein intake.

    d. more / breastmilk has a higher caloric density than formula.

37. With respect to a breastfed child, complete weaning that is delayed until the child is about 2½ years old is

    a. a sign of an emotionally needy mother.

    b. considerably longer than the usual age at which infants wean themselves.

    c. harmful to the well-being of the infant.

    d. similar to the minimum age of weaning among other primates.

Discussion Questions

1. What are the various states of arousal in an infant? Which state is optimal for breastfeeding? Why is this so?

2. What is the relationship between sleeping with an infant and infant night waking? Prolonged breast-feeding? What physiology underlies any advantage to night breastfeeds?

3. What reflexes are present during a healthy infant's first few months? What effect, if any, do they have on breastfeeding?

4. Does the addition of solid foods make a young infant (less than 4 months old) more likely to gain weight more quickly? Sleep through the night? Explain the physiology underlying your response.

5. What does the addition of table foods to a 4-month-old infant's diet do to maternal milk volumes? What will happen to milk volumes if solids are delayed until 6 or 7 months?

6. Can solids be added in such a way that they do not decrease breastmilk intake? If so, how?

7. Can breastfeeding toddlers develop tooth decay? Why or why not? What mechanisms are in operation?

8. What are standard immunizations recommended (in the United States, by the Centers for Disease Control and Prevention) for young children?
   - What vaccines have recently been added to the schedule?
   - On what schedule are they recommended to be given? Is meeting the schedule important?
   - Should breastfed infants be on the same immunization schedule as formula-fed infants?
   - What aspects of immunization are controversial? What will you recommend to parents of an infant or young child?
   - What are the benefits and risks of vaccines that contain attenuated live virus? That contain inactivated or "killed" virus?

The Ill Child: Breastfeeding Implications

Introduction

Can children breastfeed if they are born with health problems or become ill? Can they be hand-fed breast-milk? Lactation consultants are expected to provide strategies that optimize breastfeeding by the compromised infant and to support the families who must cope with emotionally draining situations. Questions in this chapter will help you to assess your understanding of this body of information and how it applies to professional practice.

IBLCE Disciplines

Information in this chapter applies to the following disciplines tested on the certification examination offered by the International Board of Lactation Consultant Examiners: E = Maternal and Infant Pathology; H = Growth Parameters and Developmental Milestones; G = Psychology, Sociology, and Anthropology; L = Techniques; 12 = General Principles.

Multiple-Choice Questions

1. The milk intake of an ill infant who is gaining poorly may be any of the following *except*

   a. inadequate, because of compositional deficiencies in his mother's milk.

   b. low, because of limited infant energy.

   c. low, because the infant guards his mouth.

   d. normal, because suckling effectiveness and appetite are normal.

2. Positioning an infant upright for breastfeeds typically will
   a. decrease the force of milk ejection because the nipple is held more forward in the mouth.
   b. decrease milk flow because the nipple usually points upward.
   c. increase alertness through stimulation of his vestibular system.
   d. tire the infant more because his jaw lacks support.

3. A good time to offer the breast to a slow-gaining breastfed infant is when the infant is _____, because then he _____.
   a. awake but quiet / will be most receptive.
   b. crying / will have his mouth wide open.
   c. fussing / probably is hungry.
   d. sleeping soundly / will be unlikely to resist.

4. Families of infants born with chronic health problems *most* appreciate advice that is
   a. accurate, so that they can develop realistic goals.
   b. detailed so that all information is on the table at once.
   c. focused on the here and now rather than future eventualities.
   d. given tactfully out of consideration for the parent's stressful situation.

5. To pace a bottle feeding for a breastfed infant who also requires supplements by bottle, a caregiver should do all of the following *except*
   a. end the feeding on baby's cue, even if milk remains in the bottle.
   b. hold the feeding bottle horizontal.
   c. tip the baby forward (bottle nipple is above horizontal) to allow the baby to rest as needed.
   d. tip the baby back (base of bottle is above horizontal) to allow the baby to rest as needed.

6. In general, a breastfed infant who receives supplements by bottle should use a bottle nipple that has all of the following characteristics *except*
   a. long enough to put tip of the nipple at the juncture of hard and soft palate.
   b. rapid flow obtained with little negative pressure.
   c. soft texture.
   d. wide base.

7. A mother who is bottle feeding her infant can retain some aspects of breastfeeding by doing all of the following *except*
   a. feeding the baby while in skin-to-skin contact.
   b. gently introducing the bottle nipple into the baby's mouth.
   c. holding the baby in the left arm for some feedings and right arm for others.
   d. maintaining eye contact with her infant.

8. Breastfeeding an infant during a painful procedure, such as a heel stick, has the effect of
   a. causing the baby to shut down.
   b. increasing heart rate.
   c. reducing crying.
   d. reducing oxygen saturation.

9. A hospital pediatric unit that encourages breastfeeding will do all of the following *except*

    a. adhere closely to a schedule of nursing procedures so the parents will have a structure to work within.

    b. allow 24-hour rooming-in of parents with their ill child.

    c. facilitate milk expression as needed.

    d. facilitate unrestricted breastfeeding.

10. A breastfed infant being prepared for surgery in the United States will be required to fast beforehand for ____ hours.

    a. 2

    b. 4

    c. 6

    d. 8

11. Following surgery, a breastfed infant may resume feeding from the breast after

    a. 12 hours.

    b. 24 hours.

    c. an initial glucose-water feeding.

    d. oral feedings are permitted.

12. One of breastfeeding's influences on child health is to reduce the risk of infection

    a. but only if the baby is exclusively breastfed.

    b. in proportion to the percentage of breastmilk taken by the infant.

    c. of minor infections but generally not major infections.

    d. principally in warm impoverished regions.

13. During an acute infectious illness, breastfed infants are characterized by all of the following *except* that they

    a. are less likely than formula-fed infants to be hospitalized.

    b. are less likely than formula-fed infants to lose weight.

    c. should continue to be breastfed insofar as the baby is able.

    d. should not be breastfed during their illness.

14. An infant is more likely to require hospitalization to treat a rotavirus infection if he has all of the following characteristics *except* that he is

    a. around other young children at home or in day care.

    b. breastfed, but by a mother who has few personal contacts outside the home.

    c. not breastfed.

    d. from a low-income home.

15. Infants with a stomach and intestinal infection (gastroenteritis) are at greater risk of _____ than older children for all of the following reasons *except* _____

    a. dehydration / less fluid may be ingested than is lost by vomiting and diarrhea.

    b. dehydration / their ratio of skin area to body volume is low.

    c. electrolyte imbalance / sodium and potassium are preferentially lost.

    d. malnutrition / food passes through the body before nutrients can be absorbed.

16. A degree of dehydration that should be treated medically is indicated by the combined appearance of all of the following *except*

    a. bowed legs.

    b. capillary refill time greater than 2 seconds.

    c. dry mucous membranes.

    d. generally ill appearance.

17. A nursing 2-year-old has gastroenteritis severe enough to cause moderate dehydration. The *best* outcome will be obtained by, for some period, feeding him oral rehydration solution and

    a. a bland diet such as banana, rice, applesauce, and toast.

    b. breastmilk and his usual table foods to maintain his nutritional status.

    c. breastmilk only, to shorten the duration of acute illness.

    d. nothing else, to give his gastrointestinal tract a rest.

18. A baby with a respiratory infection can *best* be helped to breastfeed more easily by use of a(n)

    a. antihistamine or decongestant to open bronchial passages.

    b. saline drops to clear matter from his eyes.

    c. upright position for breastfeeds.

    d. warm-air vaporizer to loosen nasal secretions.

19. A breastfed infant in whom an ear infection has developed will likely be more comfortable if he is fed _____, because _____.

    a. at longer intervals for longer times / so doing minimizes handling of the baby.

    b. in a supine position / the ill infant expends less energy.

    c. in an upright position / it minimizes discomfort in the middle ear.

    d. only when he will not accept a pacifier / the pacifier better calms the infant.

20. Excessively low muscle tone (hypotonia) can express itself in a breastfeeding infant by

    a. an easily stimulated gag reflex.

    b. complete seal of lips on the breast.

    c. consistent tongue peristalsis.

    d. generation of little negative pressure during suck.

21. Excessively high muscle tone (hypertonia) can express itself in a breastfeeding infant by

    a. a cupped tongue.

    b. a wide gape before latching onto the breast.

    c. arching of the back.

    d. breast falling to the back of the infant's mouth.

22. Both hypotonic and hypertonic infants are likely to obtain more milk at the breast if the mother uses

    a. a thin silicone nipple shield.

    b. a tube-feeding device at the breast.

    c. a tube-feeding device on a finger.

    d. breast shells.

23. Infants born with Down syndrome are likely to
    a. be hypertonic.
    b. be unable to breastfeed.
    c. grow at the same rate as healthy infants.
    d. protrude their tongue.

24. A breastfeeding neonate who has congenital heart disease is likely to
    a. begin a feeding with vigorous suckling.
    b. breathe slowly during feedings.
    c. maintain a pink flush to the skin.
    d. nurse at a consistent pace throughout the feeding.

25. The *best* predictor of duration of any breastfeeding by an infant with heart defects is the
    a. infant's birth weight.
    b. innate breastfeeding ability of the infant.
    c. mother's determination to continue.
    d. severity of the defect.

26. As compared with formula-fed infants with heart disease, breastfed infants with heart disease
    a. expend more energy during feedings.
    b. gain somewhat more weight.
    c. have higher oxygen saturation.
    d. have weight gain inversely related to the severity of the defect.

27. A breastfed infant with moderate or severe congenital heart disease commonly gains weight _____, because _____.
    a. poorly or not at all / of a high respiratory rate.
    b. poorly or not at all / of a slow heart rate.
    c. slowly but steadily / breastmilk is metabolized with almost no waste.
    d. slowly but steadily / his extra energy expenditure is only slightly higher than normal.

28. A breastfed baby with congenital heart disease is likely to feed better in a position that
    a. extends his torso.
    b. flexes his knees.
    c. hyperextends his neck.
    d. tips his chin down.

29. Most infants born with a cleft of lip or palate or with Pierre Robin sequence
    a. gain weight well with exclusive direct breastfeeding once a good position is determined.
    b. obtain little benefit from breastfeeding because milk easily strays from the oral cavity.
    c. require smaller volumes of milk to meet metabolic needs.
    d. risk failure to thrive with exclusive direct breastfeeding.

30. A small, isolated cleft of the soft palate in a breastfed infant is

    a. an extremely rare type of cleft.

    b. associated with a placid infant.

    c. commonly prevents the infant from generating full suction while nursing.

    d. of little concern because the breast fills the infant's mouth.

31. As compared with normal infants, those infants born with cleft of the lip are at _____ risk of poor mother-infant attachment *principally* because _____.

    a. greater / feedings give so little satisfaction to the mother.

    b. greater / most mothers finds the infant's appearance unattractive.

    c. less / hospital social workers are at hand to help parents cope.

    d. less / maternal protective instincts are strongly elicited.

32. Immediately following surgery to correct a cleft lip, a breastfed infant should *best* begin feeding by taking milk from a

    a. bottle containing breastmilk.

    b. breast.

    c. dropper or syringe.

    d. small, soft cup.

33. Breastmilk feedings reduce the risk of ear infections in infants with clefts or Pierre Robin sequence during the interval of

    a. about 4 months after birth.

    b. any breastfeeding.

    c. any breastfeeding and beyond complete weaning.

    d. exclusive breastfeeding.

34. A baby born with cleft lip (not palate) can usually breastfeed if

    a. a maternal finger is used to help seal the cleft as he latches onto the breast.

    b. he is interested, but that is the exception rather than the rule.

    c. he is swaddled.

    d. his cleft is positioned in the upper quadrants of the breast.

35. Normal weight gain in an infant born with cleft palate (not lip) is extremely difficult, because the infant typically has difficulty doing all of the following *except*

    a. generating the negative pressure that helps expel milk from the breast.

    b. keeping milk out of his nostrils.

    c. maintaining the breast positioned inside his mouth.

    d. sealing his lips on the breast.

36. Breastmilk intake by an infant with cleft palate can be maximized by positioning the infant so that he is

    a. cradled.

    b. prone on his mother's chest.

    c. side-lying.

    d. upright.

37. An infant with Pierre Robin sequence is unlikely to feed well at the breast because of all of the following *except*

    a. associated cleft lip.

    b. difficulty maintaining his airway.

    c. small receded chin.

    d. tongue positioned well back in the mouth.

38. Infants who regurgitate quantities of milk each day

    a. are most content when placed on their left side.

    b. except for a small minority are healthy and normal.

    c. have an especially relaxed upper esophageal sphincter.

    d. rarely outgrow this problem.

39. Thickening milk—to be fed by bottle to an infant with gastroesophageal reflux—with cereal is a _____ idea because _____.

    a. good / thickened feedings reduce or eliminate coughing by the infant.

    b. good / thicker stomach contents stick better to the walls of the esophagus and are not spit out of the mouth.

    c. poor / enzymes in breastmilk quickly break down the thickening agents.

    d. poor / the number of reflux episodes typically increases.

40. Gastroesophageal reflux episodes can be minimized by all of the following *except* _____ because _____.

    a. feeding at shorter intervals / milk volumes ingested will be smaller.

    b. feeding on one breast per feeding / it transfers more high-calorie hindmilk.

    c. positioning the baby upright for feedings / it reduces pressure on his abdomen.

    d. putting him to sleep on his right side / it reduces pressure on his esophagus.

41. The projectile vomiting that commonly accompanies uncorrected pyloric stenosis may lead to all of the following *except*

    a. dehydration.

    b. electrolyte imbalance.

    c. lack of infant interest in feeding.

    d. severe weight loss in the infant.

42. After surgery to correct pyloric stenosis, breastfeeding may resume

    a. after a 24-hour fast to allow the incision site to begin healing.

    b. after glucose-water feedings are well tolerated.

    c. by using brief breastfeeds gradually lengthened during the first 72 hours after surgery.

    d. with breastfeeds as long and often as the baby desires.

43. To maximally reduce the phenylalanine (PHE) load in infants born with phenylketonuria, these infants should be fed
    a. a prescribed amount of PHE-free formula, combined with breastmilk.
    b. exclusively breastmilk.
    c. exclusively low-phenylalanine manufactured baby milk.
    d. standard infant formula combined with phenylalanine-free manufactured baby milk.

44. Infants with phenylketonuria whose diet includes some breastmilk, as compared with similar infants who receive no breastmilk, have been shown to score _____ on test of intelligence.
    a. 3 or 4 points higher.
    b. 3 or 4 points lower.
    c. about 12 points higher.
    d. about the same.

45. Which of the following conditions contraindicates any breastfeeding?
    a. Celiac disease
    b. Chylothorax
    c. Cystic fibrosis
    d. Galactosemia

46. Jaundice in the newborn infant may be caused by all of the following *except*
    a. diabetes (type 1).
    b. galactosemia.
    c. hypothyroidism.
    d. rapid hemolysis.

47. Celiac disease in an at-risk infant is best delayed if the mother continues breastfeeding
    a. as long as possible combined with early introduction of solids.
    b. as long as possible combined with late introduction of solids.
    c. exclusively only a few weeks, then introducing formula and solids.
    d. exclusively only briefly, then introducing formula but delaying solids.

48. As compared with infant formula, breastmilk promotes growth of infants born with cystic fibrosis because it
    a. contains much more milk lipase, which aids the absorption of fats.
    b. increases the infant's appetite, so more milk is consumed.
    c. promotes absorption of vitamin D and calcium, which increase rate of linear growth.
    d. remains in the infant's stomach longer, allowing more nutrients to be absorbed.

49. Neonates who show no adverse reaction to a feeding of cow-based manufactured milk in the hospital
    a. are too young to develop allergic reactions.
    b. may express allergic symptoms if they ingest cow milk later.
    c. will never be allergic to cow milk.
    d. will not develop any allergic reaction if all subsequent feedings are cow milk-based formulas.

50. Allergic reactions in an exclusively breastfed baby are most likely a response to
    a. breastmilk itself.
    b. fats in the breastmilk, which reflect maternal diet.
    c. foreign proteins in the breastmilk.
    d. inhalants or topical substances.

51. Infants may be sensitized to allergens in all of the following ways *except*
    a. before birth, across the placenta.
    b. ingestion of an allergenic food in hospital or daycare.
    c. feeds of a nonsoy-based hypoallergenic formula.
    d. while breastfeeding, owing to foreign proteins in the milk.

52. Transient lactase deficiency in a breastfed infant's intestinal brush border may be preceded by all of the following *except*
    a. administration of analgesics.
    b. administration of antibiotics to the infant.
    c. feeding (at each nursing) from both breasts of a mother with an abundant milk supply.
    d. gastrointestinal illness in the infant.

Discussion Questions

1. How might a mother who suspects family allergies to certain foods or groups of foods reduce the risk of atopic illness in a child? What can she do before the new baby is born? What can she do after the baby is born?

2. What is the difference between food allergy, food sensitivity, and food intolerance? How does breastfeeding affect each?

3. What are five foods that are associated with allergic reactions in infants and young children? What is the offending molecule in the food?

4. What are advantages—to the infant, family, and healthcare system—of early repair of cleft lip?

5. What is the relationship between breastfeeding and upper respiratory infection in infants? Breastfeeding and lower respiratory infection? What accounts for any difference?

6. What infant illnesses are contraindications to exclusive breastfeeding or to even partial breastfeeding? What physiology underlies these illnesses?

7. As compared with the fasting period before and after surgery for infants fed manufactured milks, how long is the fasting period—both before and after surgery—for a breastfed infant? How can a mother comfort her infant during this fasting interval?

8. How does each of the following conditions affect oral feedings in general and breastfeeding in particular?
   • Choanal atresia
   • Cleft palate
   • Tracheoesophageal fistula
   • Pyloric stenosis
   • Imperforate anus
   • Esophageal reflux

9. What main points would you, a lactation consultant, make to the staff of an emergency room who must care temporarily for a breastfeeding mother or a breastfeeding infant?

10. How would you help and comfort a breastfeeding mother, physically and emotionally, whose young infant has died? Discuss at least three ways.

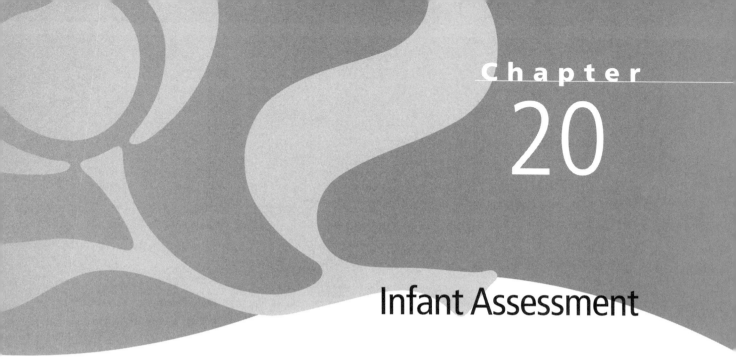

Infant Assessment

Introduction

The new baby's contribution to bringing in his mother's milk supply cannot be overemphasized. An evaluation of the infant's motor abilities, reflexes, and neurobehavioral states will suggest specific strategies for the lactation consultant to use as she helps the mother initiate breastfeeding. Questions in this chapter will help you to assess your understanding of this body of information and how it applies to professional practice.

IBLCE Disciplines

Information in this chapter applies to the following disciplines tested on the certification examination offered by the International Board of Lactation Consultant Examiners: A = Maternal and Infant Anatomy; B = Maternal and Infant Normal Physiology and Endocrinology; H = Growth Parameters and Developmental Milestones; L = Techniques; 12 = General Principles.

Multiple-Choice Questions

1. A complete assessment of a newborn infant evaluates all of the following *except*
   a. ability to feed.
   b. gestational age.
   c. infant's focal distance.
   d. maternal perinatal history.

2. As applied to a newborn, the New Ballard Score evaluates _____ in order to estimate gestational age.
   a. ability to coordinate suckle, swallow, and breathe
   b. infant birth date against mother's estimated due date
   c. infant birthweight against standard intrauterine-growth charts
   d. six physical and six neuromuscular signs

3. An infant's physical and neuromuscular maturity at birth is influenced by all of the following *except*
   a. birth order.
   b. date of mother's last menstrual period.
   c. inborn genetic disorders.
   d. maternal chronic illness.

4. An infant is considered full term if he is born between _____ and _____ weeks gestational age.
   a. 36 / 40
   b. 37 / 41
   c. 37 / 42
   d. 38 / 42

5. A newborn is born at 38 weeks gestation and with a birth weight below the 10th percentile on the intrauterine-growth curve. How would he be would be classified on the basis of size?
   a. Appropriate for gestational age (AGA)
   b. Low birth weight (LBW)
   c. Small for gestational age (SGA)
   d. Very low birth weight (VLBW)

6. An infant classified as low birthweight (LBW) weighs between about _____ and _____ pounds at birth.
   a. 3 / 5
   b. 4 / 6
   c. 4 / 7
   d. 5 / 7

7. A baby girl born at 36 weeks gestation and 7½ pounds is classified as
   a. appropriate for gestational age.
   b. premature, according to age.
   c. premature only if labia majora do not cover labia minora.
   d. term, according to weight.

8. Infants who breastfeed effectively typically do all of the following *except*
   a. drop the nipple while they pause between suckling bursts.
   b. grasp the nipple firmly.
   c. suckle rhythmically in bursts.
   d. turn their mouth to the mother's nipple when brought to breast.

9. Audible swallowing by a neonate who is at the breast likely indicates that
   a. lactogenesis I has just occurred.
   b. milk is being transferred.
   c. the baby is less than 3 days old.
   d. the baby's tongue is too far back in his mouth.

10. A 2-day-old infant who is rooting typically

    a. lifts his tongue to the roof of his mouth.

    b. makes licking movements.

    c. purses his lips.

    d. turns his head toward a stimulus.

11. An infant who latches firmly onto the breast

    a. has a tonic bite.

    b. has his lower lip turned in.

    c. is probably creasing his mother's nipple.

    d. retains the breast during pauses in suckling.

12. During swallowing, an infant well latched onto the breast also

    a. depresses the back of his tongue.

    b. drops and then raises his lower jaw.

    c. flares his nares to obtain oxygen.

    d. retracts his cheeks.

13. A breastfeeding-assessment tool can be used for all of the following purposes *except* as a(n)

    a. method of documenting the baby's feeding ability.

    b. outcome measure in research on breastfeeding.

    c. record from which breastmilk intake can be calculated.

    d. tool to teach the mother about her baby's breastfeeding abilities.

14. The success of the LATCH breastfeeding-assessment tool in predicting who would still be breastfeeding at 6 weeks postpartum relies principally on which item?

    a. Audible swallowing

    b. How much help mother needs to position infant

    c. How well infant latches onto the breast

    d. Mother's nipple comfort

15. Of the breastfeeding assessment tools listed below, which has been shown to have the highest reliability and validity?

    a. Infant Breastfeeding Assessment Tool (IBFAT)

    b. LATCH Assessment Tool

    c. Mother-Baby Assessment Tool (MBA)

    d. Via Christi Breastfeeding Assessment Tool

16. Of the breastfeeding-assessment tools listed below, which has been shown to *best* predict the amount of breastmilk ingested by an infant?

    a. LATCH Assessment Tool

    b. Mother-Baby Assessment Tool (MBA)

    c. Preterm Infant Breastfeeding Behavior Scale (PIBBS)

    d. Via Christi Breastfeeding Assessment Tool

17. Of the various aspects of breastfeeding that assessment tools measure, which aspect *best* predicts milk intake?

    a. Audible swallowing

    b. Lips flanged outward

    c. Maternal nipple comfort

    d. Visible swallowing

18. Putting a baby to breast within the first 30 minutes after birth is _____, because _____.

    a. not necessary / the baby will soon fall into a deep sleep and doesn't need the calories.

    b. poor / the baby needs to recover from labor and delivery and shouldn't be expending energy unnecessarily.

    c. recommended / so doing will hasten the onset of lactogenesis II.

    d. recommended / the baby (if unmedicated) will actively root and latch.

19. After an initial awake-and-alert phase, a newborn falls into a deep sleep, during which

    a. body temperature stabilizes.

    b. heart rate decreases.

    c. production of mucus increases.

    d. respiratory rate increases.

20. Most newborns will have passed their first meconium stool within the first _____ hours after birth.

    a. 4

    b. 8

    c. 16

    d. 24

21. The skin of an infant born at 35 weeks gestational age typically will show

    a. blood vessels visible on the trunk.

    b. dry or peeling hands and feet.

    c. flaking skin in deep creases.

    d. prominent vernix caseosa.

22. As a function of ethnicity, the native color of a newborn's skin on day 1 may be any of the following colors *except*

    a. pink.

    b. pink with olive tinge.

    c. tan.

    d. yellowish to white.

23. Neonatal skin that quickly regains its original shape after being gently pinched typically indicates

    a. adequate interstitial fluid in the skin.

    b. excessive fetal weight gain in the third trimester.

    c. that the infant is "late premature."

    d. that the infant requires more fluid.

24. A young infant's anterior fontanelle
    a. closes between 2 and 4 months of age.
    b. depresses when the infant coughs.
    c. has a triangular shape.
    d. is sunken when the infant is dehydrated.

25. A neonate's visual abilities enable him to
    a. converge his eyes to focus on nearby objects.
    b. focus on objects about 20 inches from his eyes.
    c. follow to the midline objects that move.
    d. respond to stationary more than to moving objects.

26. In a healthy term neonate, a familiar voice typically will elicit
    a. an eyeblink.
    b. immediate initiation of or increase in movement of arms and legs.
    c. steady gaze at the speaker.
    d. wrinkling of the brow.

27. The nose of a full-term newborn
    a. cannot be compressed on one nostril without compromising the infant's air supply.
    b. contains sufficient cartilage to avoid being misshapen at birth.
    c. drains mucus for the first few days after birth.
    d. may be the terminus of a cleft lip or palate.

28. The mouth of a normal, healthy term neonate contains _____ that _____.
    a. a gum ridge / confines the tongue when the mouth is open.
    b. a tongue / fits easily behind the gumline when his mouth is closed.
    c. buccal pads / are thin but which thicken rapidly as breastfeeding progresses.
    d. mucous membranes / are relatively dry to give the mouth more traction on the breast.

29. A tight lingual frenulum in the infant may be associated with
    a. creased but comfortable maternal nipples.
    b. inability to extend the tongue beyond the lower gum ridge.
    c. smooth philtrum in the center of the upper lip.
    d. very short jaw excursions during breastfeeding.

30. Noticeable drooling by a neonate is a questionable sign that may indicate all of the following *except*
    a. difficulty swallowing.
    b. obstruction in the esophagus.
    c. obstruction in the pharynx.
    d. overactive salivary glands.

31. A healthy term neonate's hard palate should be
    a. covered with pronounced rugae that help hold the breast in place.
    b. gently arched with a small cleft in the soft palate.
    c. smooth and contain a high central bubble.
    d. smooth, gently arched, and intact.

32. As compared with the circumference of his chest, the circumference of a neonate's head
    a. is nearly always exactly the same.
    b. is slightly (about 2 cm) larger.
    c. is slightly (about 2 cm) smaller.
    d. may be either larger or smaller; there is no consistent difference.

33. A neonate whose chest retracts while he breathes is
    a. asking to be put to the breast, where he will breathe more regularly.
    b. hungry and should be put to the breast.
    c. overly excited; swaddle to calm him before trying to breastfeed.
    d. working hard to breathe and is unlikely to breastfeed well.

34. Bowel sounds usually can be heard within____ hour(s) after birth.
    a. 1
    b. 12
    c. 24
    d. 36

35. Drops of bloody discharge in the vaginal opening of a neonate is *most* likely to indicate a
    a. breech birth.
    b. response to high maternal estrogen concentrations during gestation.
    c. response to high maternal progesterone concentrations during gestation.
    d. rupture of small capillaries during labor.

36. In the first week postpartum, pink or red stains in the diaper owing to uric acid crystals are a consequence of
    a. at least one cow-milk feeding.
    b. at least one soy-milk feeding.
    c. excess intake of foremilk after lactogenesis II.
    d. poor hydration.

37. During the first week postpartum, a breastfed newborn's stools change color as follows
    a. black, greenish brown, green.
    b. black, greenish brown, mustard.
    c. brownish black, yellow, green.
    d. greenish black, tan, brown.

38. The sleep–wake states in which a newborn breastfeeds most effectively are _____ and _____.

    a. deep sleep / quiet alert.

    b. drowsy / quiet alert.

    c. quiet alert / active alert.

    d. quiet sleep / drowsy.

39. A newborn who arches and grimaces is

    a. energetic and ready to interact with others.

    b. hungry and ready to feed.

    c. overstimulated and needs rest.

    d. sleepy and ready for the crib.

40. Early cues that a baby is hungry include all of the following *except* that the baby

    a. brings his hands to his mouth.

    b. cries.

    c. extends his tongue.

    d. turns his head to the side.

Discussion Questions

1. Describe the normal range of vital signs (temperature, pulse, respirations) in a newborn.

2. Describe three features of infant anatomy that are directly related to the neonate's ability to suckle. How could early assessment of these features help prevent breastfeeding failure?

3. Name three breastfeeding assessment tools. Which tool do you think is best to use in clinical practice? Why do you think so?

4. Complete a physical assessment of a breastfeeding baby less than 6 weeks old. Describe the main physical and behavioral features of the infant as you progress through the assessment. Are the features you describe appropriate for the infant's age?

5. Describe sleep–wake states in which an infant is most receptive to latching onto the breast.

6. Practice using the New Ballard Score to determine the gestational age of a newborn baby.

7. Describe the same (as in previous question) neonate's mouth size and symmetry of shape, and tongue placement when he is at rest, is crying, and is well latched onto the breast. Describe normal characteristics of each.

8. A child's behavior while feeding at the breast changes as the child grows and develops. Demonstrate how a 2-week-old child behaves while he is breastfeeding. Then, demonstrate how a 15-month-old child behaves while he is breastfeeding.

9. Name at least one breastfeeding risk factor associated with an infant who is small for gestational age.

10. A preterm baby is one who is born before how many weeks? Does 1 or 2 weeks of prematurity affect a baby's breastfeeding abilities? If so, what is the effect? What assistance should a lactation consultant be prepared to offer?

Chapter 21

Fertility, Sexuality, and Contraception During Lactation

Introduction

Sexuality, fertility, contraception, and lactation mutually interact in both physiological and psychological ways. A lactation consultant must understand these interactions before she can respond to inquiries about sexual relations and contraception during the breastfeeding interval. Questions in this chapter will help you to assess your understanding of this body of information and how it applies to professional practice.

IBLCE Disciplines

Information in this chapter applies to the following disciplines tested on the certification examination offered by the International Board of Lactation Consultant Examiners: B = Maternal and Infant Normal Physiology and Endocrinology; I = Interpretation of Research.

Multiple-Choice Questions

1. It is thought that suckling interferes with the secretion of gonadotopin-releasing hormone, which in turn leads to secretion of insufficient _____ to cause ovulation.

    a. estrogen

    b. progestin

    c. prolactin

    d. thyroid

2. After childbirth but before a woman's menses return, she will ovulate

    a. at least twice.

    b. never.

    c. no more than one time.

    d. several times.

3. All of the following influence suppression of ovulation, but only _____ can be relatively easily measured.

    a. number of feedings per day

    b. satiety after feedings

    c. suckling intensity

    d. volume of milk obtained

4. A mother who breastfeeds at least seven times daily will reliably prevent ovulation.

    a. False, even in exclusively breastfeeding well-nourished mothers

    b. False, except in exclusively breastfeeding undernourished mothers

    c. True, but only in exclusively breastfeeding well-nourished mothers

    d. True, in all mothers after 6 months postpartum

5. The link between supplementing a breastfed infant and return of menses is that

    a. breastmilk loses much of its nutritive value after menses return and the infant must be supplemented.

    b. most supplemented infants are older than 6 months, when menses will return shortly in any case.

    c. the amount of suckling falls below some threshold needed to suppress ovulation.

    d. the imminent return of menses reduces milk volume, so that the infant needs supplements.

6. Adding any nonbreastmilk food to an infant's diet _____ precede(s) return of menses _____.

    a. is likely to / if it is added after several months of exclusive breastfeeding.

    b. nearly always / in breastfeeding women in general.

    c. nearly always / in undernourished women.

    d. will likely / if the additional food replaces one or more breastfeedings.

7. The length of lactation amenorrhea while breastfeeding any one child _____ the length of amenorrhea while breastfeeding a subsequent child.

    a. bears no relation to

    b. decreases with each successive child

    c. increases with each successive child

    d. is roughly similar to

8. Vaginal bleeding in a breastfeeding woman during the first few weeks postpartum indicates that she has

    a. normal postpartum bleeding and fertility has not yet returned.

    b. ovulated and is fertile.

    c. resumed sexual relations too soon.

    d. returned to menstrual cycling but did not ovulate beforehand.

9. The Bellagio Consensus states that exclusive breastfeeding during the first _____ months postpartum, in the absence of vaginal bleeding after day 56 postpartum, provides about _____ percent protection against pregnancy.

    a. 3 / 75

    b. 4 / 75

    c. 6 / 15

    d. 6 / 98

10. Breastfeeding exclusively for 6 months
    a. depletes the mother's body stores to a harmful degree.
    b. is nutritionally inadequate for the infant.
    c. normally produces optimal growth in the infant.
    d. provides adequate weight gain but stunts the infant somewhat.

11. Low progesterone concentrations in the blood may be associated with feelings of
    a. increased energy.
    b. optimism.
    c. relaxation.
    d. vulnerability.

12. Maternal use of a topical estrogen crème to relieve vaginal dryness may also lead to a
    a. decrease in milk volume.
    b. disruption of night-time sleep.
    c. perianal skin rash similar to a *Candida* rash.
    d. postponement of ovulation.

13. One can conclude from various studies of the effect of breastfeeding on a sexual relationship that breastfeeding typically _____ coital frequency and enjoyment.
    a. decreases
    b. has no consistently predictable effect on
    c. has no effect on
    d. increases

14. Categories of contraceptive methods for lactating women, in order from most preferred to least preferred, are _____, _____, and _____.
    a. estrogen-containing / progestin only / nonhormonal.
    b. progestin only / nonhormonal / estrogen containing.
    c. nonhormonal / estrogen containing / progestin only.
    d. nonhormonal / progestin only / estrogen containing.

15. Counseling about contraceptive methods is ideally provided _____, with follow-up _____.
    a. after 6 weeks postpartum / verifying that breastfeeding is going well.
    b. after hospital discharge / at the 6-week visit.
    c. before delivery / postpartum, timed to match the method chosen.
    d. immediately after delivery / within the first 2 weeks postpartum.

16. The lactation amenorrhea method of contraception can be relied upon during the
    a. entire course of breastfeeding.
    b. first 6 months postpartum.
    c. first 9 months postpartum.
    d. interval in which the infant is taking at least three breastfeeds per day.

17. A breastfeeding mother using lactation amenorrhea for contraception does not need to begin another method of contraception when she begins to

    a. engage in sexual relations more than twice per week.

    b. enter her 7th month postpartum.

    c. feed her infant nonbreastmilk foods that replace a breastfeeding.

    d. have vaginal bleeding not related to postpartum lochia flow.

18. Nonhormonal intrauterine devices, when they are used in lactating women, tend to

    a. be retained more commonly if inserted during the 6-week postpartum period.

    b. be retained more commonly if inserted immediately after delivery of the placenta.

    c. increase the leukocyte content of breastmilk.

    d. markedly increase the risk of uterine perforation.

19. Estrogen and progestin in hormonal contraceptives used in the early months postpartum are of _____ concern, because _____.

    a. considerable / large percentages are excreted in breastmilk.

    b. little or no / the fetus is exposed to much higher concentrations of other hormones in utero.

    c. no / they have no effect on milk secretion or release.

    d. some / small amounts are excreted in breastmilk, but the infant metabolizes them poorly.

20. The earliest time recommended for a breastfeeding mother to begin use of a progestin-only contraceptive is

    a. about 6-months postpartum.

    b. about 6-weeks postpartum.

    c. after the infant has begun to take nonbreastmilk foods.

    d. as soon as milk has matured.

21. Progestin-only contraceptives, with the possible exception of progestin injected within the first few weeks, _____ associated with _____.

    a. are / delayed development of infant motor skills.

    b. are / delayed infant growth.

    c. are not / diminished milk secretion.

    d. are not / irregular bleeding.

22. The physiological trigger for the initiation of abundant milk production is

    a. secretion of a high concentration of prolactin.

    b. secretion of luteinizing hormone.

    c. withdrawal of estrogen.

    d. withdrawal of progesterone.

23. A breastfeeding woman who wishes to begin using an estrogen-containing contraceptive by 4-weeks postpartum probably should be _____ because it _____.

    a. discouraged / diminishes the oxytocin response and thus weakens milk ejection.

    b. discouraged / increases risk of maternal thrombosis in the postpartum period.

    c. encouraged / effectively prevents a new conception.

    d. encouraged / increases maternal milk volume.

Discussion   Questions

1. What are the relationships among the following?
   - Contraception
   - Fertility
   - Sexuality
   - Lactation

2. Name examples of a hormonal contraceptive, a permanent nonhormonal contraceptive, and a non-permanent, nonhormonal contraceptive. What is the effect of each type of contraceptive on breast-feeding?

3. For women in a developing region, what are the advantages and disadvantages of each type of con-traceptive described above? Are the advantages and disadvantages the same for women living in in-dustrialized regions?

4. What criteria must be met for the lactational amenorrhea method of contraception to function optimally?

5. What is the effect of infant suckling on continued milk production? On inhibition of ovulation? Is total minutes of suckling per 24 hours the only consideration, or does spacing throughout the 24 hours have an effect too?

6. When menses return, is the lactation amenorrhea method of contraception still sufficient? Why or why not?

7. What roles do gonadotropin-releasing hormone and luteinizing hormone play during the normal menstrual cycle of a nonlactating woman? Are concentrations of these hormones different in a lac-tating and a nonlactating woman? If so, in what way?

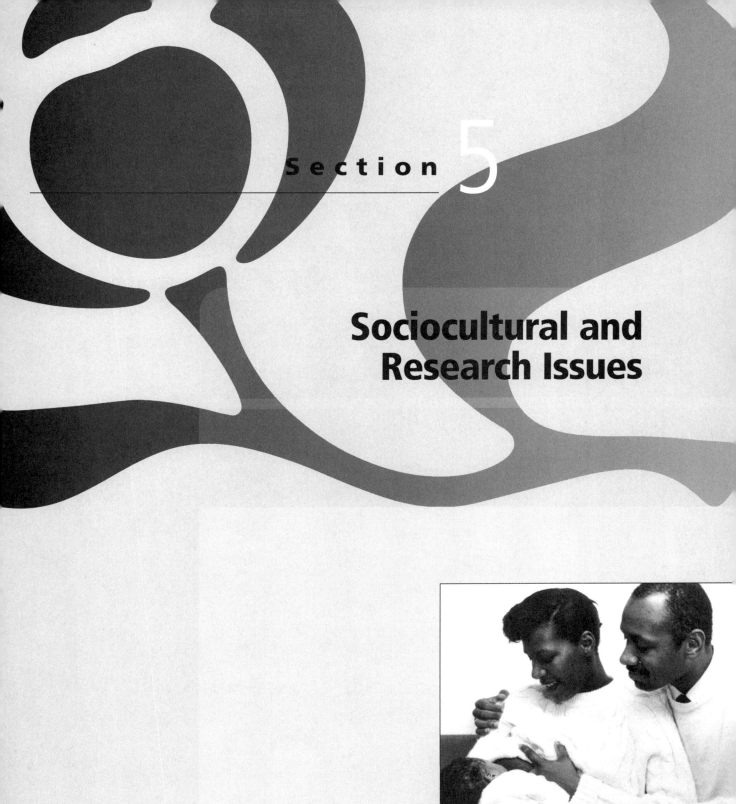

Section 5

Sociocultural and
Research Issues

Research, Theory, and Lactation

Introduction

If we are to make the best possible recommendations about breastfeeding management, we must have the best possible information about the physical, emotional, and social milieus of breastfeeding. How is that information obtained and analyzed? Lactation consultants must understand how to interpret findings reported in the published literature on breastfeeding and how to decide if the conclusions are clinically relevant. Questions in this chapter will help you to assess your understanding of this body of information and how it applies to professional practice.

IBLCE Disciplines

Information in this chapter applies to the following discipline tested on the certification examination offered by the International Board of Lactation Consultant Examiners: I = Interpretation of Research.

Multiple-Choice Questions

1. One goal of qualitative research is
   a. detailed descriptions of people's experiences.
   b. determining the nature of independent variables.
   c. gathering data that test a previously developed hypothesis.
   d. investigating a broadly defined topic in greater detail.

2. A report titled "The Experience of Living with an Incessantly Crying Infant" is *most* likely to be an example of which research method?

   a. Correlational

   b. Grounded theory

   c. Participatory action

   d. Phenomenology

3. Grounded theory refers to a method that

   a. describes behaviors influencing a person's perceived ability to complete a task.

   b. explains actions as a function of the intention to perform the action.

   c. generates theories based on people's interpretations of their own experiences.

   d. is used to understand beliefs and practices within a particular culture.

4. Correlational studies examine

   a. only variables that vary directly with each other.

   b. only variables that vary inversely with each other.

   c. qualitative data in narrative form.

   d. relationships among the variables studied.

5. One requirement of an experimental study is that

   a. at least one independent and one dependent variable are evaluated.

   b. data are collected at the "ordinal" level.

   c. no intervention is used.

   d. study subjects may come from a convenience sample.

6. A research design is considered to be quasi-experimental if it

   a. applies ethnographic techniques to a randomized group in which confounders have been eliminated.

   b. evaluates an intervention and eliminates confounders but does not randomize subjects.

   c. gathers data by use of a questionnaire with an established validity and reliability.

   d. gathers data by use of an untested questionnaire.

7. A descriptive study typically is undertaken when a topic of interest

   a. can be completed without face-to-face interviews.

   b. can be investigated solely by observational techniques.

   c. is little understood because of lack of information.

   d. will require little statistical manipulation in order to make sense of the data.

8. Observational research relies upon information gathered through

   a. interviews of people who have observed a given behavior of interest.

   b. reports of close associates who have observed a person of interest.

   c. reports of investigators who have observed a behavior of interest.

   d. self-report questionnaires of people who have observed a behavior of interest.

9. While planning a research study, an investigator must
   a. avoid reading previous reports on the topic so as not to be influenced by their conclusions.
   b. determine what research methods to use.
   c. obtain access to subjects who are willing to participate without knowing the goals of the research.
   d. wait to state a hypothesis until trends begin to emerge from the data.

10. The factor believed to cause changes in an outcome variable is called a(n) _____ variable.
    a. independent
    b. intervention
    c. quasi-dependent
    d. superior

11. Factors that the investigator did not eliminate, but which still influence the outcome of a study, are called _____ variables.
    a. confounding
    b. grounded
    c. recruited
    d. shadow

12. A research hypothesis typically
    a. limits research to those studies for which data will be manipulated statistically.
    b. serves as the starting point of a qualitative study.
    c. states expected relationships between variables in a given population.
    d. sums up the outcome of an experimental or correlational study.

13. When a null hypothesis is written, it is phrased to say that the independent
    a. and dependent variables are not related in a statistically significant manner.
    b. and dependent variables are related in a statistically significantly manner.
    c. variable is the only variable likely to affect the dependent variable.
    d. variable will cause no change in the dependent variable.

14. Operational definitions explicitly describe how
    a. equipment used in the study is to be operated and maintained.
    b. terms used for each major variable in the study are defined.
    c. the experiment will operate—such as number of subjects and length of follow-up.
    d. tools (such as questionnaires that will be used in the study) were developed.

15. The *most* important reason that studies of the relationship between breastfeeding and infant health may disagree is that
    a. breastfeeding may be defined differently in different studies.
    b. mothers of tracked infants may produce differing amounts of milk.
    c. the length of time that infants are tracked may differ.
    d. the number of infants tracked may differ.

16. A person participating in medical research must
    a. agree to participate for the entire duration of the study.
    b. agree to allow responses to link to at least some personal identifiers.
    c. be told something about the study.
    d. receive a full explanation of the treatment to be received.

17. An investigator can meet her obligation to obtain informed consent from a prospective subject by fully describing the study _____ and receiving a(n) _____ consent.
    a. in writing / oral.
    b. in writing / written.
    c. orally / oral.
    d. orally / written.

18. Probability sampling is used when
    a. few subjects are available, and it is probable that nearly all must be recruited.
    b. investigators recruit subjects for a qualitative study.
    c. investigators recruit subjects who are most probable to demonstrate the hypothesis being tested.
    d. subjects are chosen at random from the entire population of possible subjects.

19. Research studies of breastfeeding dyads are *most* apt to follow which sampling technique?
    a. Convenience
    b. Simple random
    c. Stratified random
    d. Systematic

20. Probability samples are preferred for _____ studies because _____.
    a. correlational / recruiting a large sample is easier.
    b. experimental / study findings are more easily generalized to larger populations.
    c. grounded theory / only a small group of subjects is needed.
    d. phenomenological / the data gathered can be analyzed statistically.

21. Statistical analysis of the data gathered by a study that ends with too few subjects may
    a. reject the null hypothesis if an inverse relationship is found between independent and outcome variables.
    b. reject the null hypothesis if a direct relationship is found between independent and outcome variables.
    c. not detect differences that in fact exist between treatment groups.
    d. not detect similarities that in fact exist between treatment groups.

22. The "reliability" of data collected during a study refers to the
    a. accuracy and consistency of equipment used to make measurements.
    b. accuracy and consistency of measurements or observations made during the investigation.
    c. appropriateness of statistical methods used to analyze the data.
    d. trustworthiness of the investigators.

23. "Validity" of a study's data-collection tools refers to the degree to which the
    a. information generated by the study is clinically useful.
    b. hypothesis tested is substantiated.
    c. method of acquiring data ensured that the data are accurate and true.
    d. null hypothesis is rejected.

24. Use of parametric statistical methods requires all of the following *except* that
    a. measurement of the dependent variable is at an interval level.
    b. only a relatively small number of subjects is needed.
    c. subjects are randomly selected.
    d. variables are normally distributed among study groups.

25. Use of nonparametric statistical methods requires all of the following *except* that
    a. large numbers of subjects are needed.
    b. measurement of variables is at the ordinal level.
    c. population parameters are unknown.
    d. variables in the sample may not be normally distributed.

26. A relative risk (or odds ratio) of _____ suggests that a group exposed to a given factor (such as exclusive breastfeeding for 3 months) has an incidence of some outcome (such as otitis media) that is _____ the incidence of the outcome in a nonexposed group.
    a. 0 / equivalent to
    b. 1 / equivalent to
    c. 5 / lower than
    d. 75 / higher than

27. Findings in a study that the investigator did not anticipate
    a. can be the basis for other research in the future.
    b. should not be published.
    c. usually appear only when the investigator looks for a relationship not specifically tested for.
    d. usually mean that the study was not properly designed at the outset.

28. In a published report, discussing the limitations of a study should
    a. be avoided because it undermines the study's credibility.
    b. emphasize the strengths of the study's design.
    c. evaluate the degree to which the study's results can be generalized.
    d. refer only to previously published work.

29. The Cochrane Collaboration compiles
    a. advocacy statements promoting public health measures such as breastfeeding.
    b. articles on basic research into anatomy and physiology.
    c. general medical articles available to anyone in the world.
    d. systematic reviews of the effect of specific interventions on human health.

Discussion Questions

1. What are the chief differences between qualitative and quantitative research? What kinds of data are produced by each type of research? What is a research question that can be investigated by each type of research?

2. What are the main differences between correlational, descriptive, and experimental research methods? What is a research question that can be investigated by each type of research?

3. What is the difference between a sample and a population? Are investigators more apt to collect information from samples or populations?

4. What are the rights of human subjects in a research study? How are those rights protected? What if the subjects are breastfeeding infants?

5. What is the difference between an independent variable, a dependent variable, and a confounding variable? How does an investigator minimize the effect of confounding variables?

6. What is an "operational" definition? Does it differ from an ordinary dictionary definition? If so, why?

7. How can a review of literature help an investigator decide whether to pursue qualitative or quantitative research?

8. What is the difference between probability sampling and nonprobability sampling as ways to obtain subjects for a study? What is an example of each sampling method?

9. What is meant by reliability and by validity? To what aspect of research does each apply?

10. What is meant by interrater reliability? Intrarater reliability? Test-retest reliability? Internal consistency? What is an example of each?

11. According to one investigator, breastfeeding duration was longest when the mother had previously breastfed, her new baby was full-term, and she was married; however, parity trended in the opposite direction. Match each factor in the left column with the appropriate descriptor in the right column, and explain your pairings.

    Marital status   Confounding variable
    Parity   Dependent (or outcome) variable
    Previous breastfeeding experience   Independent variable
    Breastfeeding duration
    Full-term infant

12. As methods of collecting data, what are the strengths and weaknesses of interviews? Field observations? Document review? In what kind of study is each method appropriately used?

13. Is a valid conclusion drawn from a well-designed research study necessarily clinically useful? How do you decide? If it is not clinically useful, how did that happen?

Breastfeeding Education

Introduction

Whether talking to one person or to an entire roomful, lactation consultants teach. It is the heart of their job. Doing so effectively requires an understanding of the characteristics of adult learners. Questions in this chapter will help you to assess your understanding of this body of information and how it applies to professional practice.

IBLCE Disciplines

Information in this chapter applies to the following discipline tested on the certification examination offered by the International Board of Lactation Consultant Examiners: M = Public Health.

Multiple-Choice Questions

1. Hospital-based breastfeeding education classes for new parents tend to increase the likelihood that attendees will have all of the following *except*

   a. favorable opinion of the hospital.

   b. knowledge of and competence in breastfeeding.

   c. preference for using another hospital for other medical needs.

   d. preference for using the same hospital for other medical needs.

2. A "teachable moment" is one in which a learner

   a. debates a topic with an instructor.

   b. experiences an "Ah-ha!" moment in which new information is understood and assimilated.

   c. feels a need for new information or skills.

   d. is confronted by a situation in which she must instruct other learners.

3. Learning incorporates all of the aspects below *except*
   a. learning facts, solving problems.
   b. mastering skills.
   c. modifying attitudes or preferences.
   d. teaching new skills to others.

4. An adult tends to learn most efficiently when the
   a. class requires active participation of students.
   b. information is sequenced in the order most useful to the instructor.
   c. students work on their own at exercises that permit focused attention.
   d. students are not directly involved in the topic, so they have some perspective on it.

5. Kinesthetic learning occurs when a learner
   a. hears material, as when attending a lecture.
   b. reads new information.
   c. touches or handles equipment or models.
   d. uses as many senses as possible to incorporate new information.

6. Adults in a class differ from children because
   a. adults are thinking primarily of others.
   b. education must be applicable to a student's practical use.
   c. the theoretical underpinnings of an action must be clearly explained.
   d. time is typically considered abundant.

7. Which of the items below *best* promotes adult education?
   a. Mesh the information presented with students' readiness to learn that information.
   b. Present information in large, comprehensive blocks.
   c. Provide specific feedback at a later date to encourage student learning.
   d. Provide take-home handouts instead of individual teaching.

8. As compared with their prepregnancy state, in the very early postpartum new mothers retain new information _____, because _____.
   a. better / her pregnancy hormonal state is resolving.
   b. better / the baby's presence sharpens perception.
   c. worse / of a hormonal mechanism related to "fight or flight."
   d. worse / she is recovering from the physical and emotional intensity of childbirth.

9. A mother usually decides how she will feed her baby
   a. around the time that she feels "quickening."
   b. during the third pregnancy trimester.
   c. long before she becomes pregnant.
   d. when she confirms her pregnancy.

10. The baby's father or grandparents _____ be encouraged to attend breastfeeding education programs because _____.

   a. should not / of the extra side conversations that typically result.

   b. should not / they commonly repeat incorrect information about breastfeeding.

   c. should / they can attend to the new baby while the mother focuses on the class.

   d. should / those people influence the mother's ability to breastfeed.

11. Before trying to teach information that the instructor thinks important, the instructor must *first*

   a. address the mother's immediate concerns.

   b. make the classroom comfortable.

   c. demonstrate her own expertise.

   d. show that she is empathetic.

12. A new mother who attends prenatal breastfeeding classes is more likely than another mother to

   a. delay the baby's first feeding at the breast.

   b. extend the period of breastfeeding.

   c. feel ambivalent about how she will feed her infant.

   d. feel overwhelmed with information.

13. A class that transmits information principally by lecture is characterized by all of the following *except*

   a. an efficient use of instructor time.

   b. an association with decreased retention of information.

   c. it makes listeners largely passive.

   d. strong listener interaction with the instructor and other listeners.

14. Retention of a newly taught skill or bit of information is increased by _____, so that learners can focus on _____.

   a. hearing it only / the instructor.

   b. hearing, seeing, and practicing / using all of their senses to learn.

   c. practicing it only / their own motor responses.

   d. seeing it only / the instructor.

15. To maximize retention of information transmitted in a class,

   a. lecture from only one or two locations in the classroom, so listeners know where to find you.

   b. describe thoroughly any tasks or skills to be learned—more than once as needed.

   c. schedule breaks after no more than 50 minutes of class.

   d. wear clothing in dark or neutral colors that are not distracting.

16. People's behavior is more likely to change if they are taught

   a. in large, structured classes, by a lecturer.

   b. in groups of 8 to 12, by an instructor.

   c. individually, by educational media such as videotapes or computer programs.

   d. individually, by an instructor.

17. Useful information to discuss in a prenatal breastfeeding class is
    a. how to clip a newborn's fingernails.
    b. how to tell the difference between pathological and physiological newborn jaundice.
    c. the benefits of putting the infant to breast within an hour after birth.
    d. treatment of a breast abscess.

18. Parent education booklets that emphasize potential problems of breastfeeding are *most* likely to
    a. appeal principally to mothers who lack a nursing or other medical background.
    b. dissuade mothers from initiating breastfeeding.
    c. give mothers a realistic view of what they may encounter.
    d. prepare mothers to recognize problems they will need medical help with.

19. As compared with parent education booklets that explain information only in narrative text, pamphlets that also use clear, accurate pictures to explain skills or concepts
    a. appear to be "talking down" to readers.
    b. distract readers from the text.
    c. increase reader recognition and recall.
    d. tend to look less authoritative.

20. Parent education booklets that emphasize the difficulty and inconvenience of breastfeeding are *most* likely to be produced by organizations that
    a. are concerned about the welfare of the mother.
    b. promote breastfeeding.
    c. sell manufactured baby milks.
    d. want to employ mothers of young infants.

21. Well-written breastfeeding education booklets
    a. are well balanced and thus favorably describe and depict bottle-feeding also.
    b. are written at a reading level useful to the readers.
    c. depict mothers of the social groups most likely to breastfeed.
    d. emphasize basic anatomy and physiology of lactation.

22. A behavioral objective typical of a continuing education program in breastfeeding management is as follows: The learner will
    a. be able to recognize three signs of infant dehydration.
    b. be able to state three early signs of infant hunger.
    c. learn how to elicit an infant gape that allows good attachment to the breast.
    d. understand the relationship between water supplements and neonatal jaundice.

23. Mother-to-mother breastfeeding support groups are intended to provide
    a. a regimen that will assure long-term breastfeeding.
    b. a regimen that will assure successful early breastfeedings.
    c. comparative descriptions of local physicians' attitudes toward breastfeeding.
    d. social and practical support for the breastfeeding mother.

Discussion Questions

1. How do adult learners differ from school-age learners? How should methods to teach about breast-feeding be modified to meet the needs of adult learners?

2. What is a teachable moment?

3. What are the differences among the visual, auditory, and kinesthetic learning modes? Pick a single breastfeeding education topic, and show how each mode might be used in teaching that topic.

4. For printed educational materials that promote breastfeeding, discuss at least three content criteria that should be met and at least three format criteria that should be met.

5. How might people in each of the following positions contribute to a program to educate hospital staff on optimal management of breastfeeding?
   - Childbirth educators
   - Dietitians
   - Lactation consultants
   - Perinatal nurses
   - Physicians
   - Volunteer breastfeeding support group leaders

6. What are modifiable maternal characteristics or situations that predict breastfeeding outcome? Which variables can be influenced by education of the mother? By education of labor and delivery room staff? How would you accomplish that?

7. Collect samples of breastfeeding education brochures designed for mothers. Evaluate the following aspects of each brochure:
   - Compliance with WHO code recommendations
   - Discussion of benefits of breastfeeding
   - Discussion of risks of feeding formula
   - Emphasis on difficulties of breastfeeding
   - Photographs or illustrations at variance with statements in the text
   - Reading level
   - Support of breastfeeding (general and specific)

8. Will you use any of the brochures evaluated in Question 7? Why or why not?

The Cultural Context of Breastfeeding

Introduction

The pull may be centrifugal or centripetal, but the norms of the culture in which we grow up remain the axis around which we rotate. Lactation consultants must understand and respect other mothers' cultural norms that concern breastfeeding and infant feeding in general. Questions in this chapter will help you to assess your understanding of this body of information and how it applies to professional practice.

IBLCE Disciplines

Information in this chapter applies to the following discipline tested on the certification examination offered by the International Board of Lactation Consultant Examiners: G = Psychology, Sociology, and Anthropology.

Multiple-Choice Questions

1. A culture
   a. does not guide decisions or actions in any predictable way.
   b. implies knowledge limited to a small, select subgroup of a population.
   c. is a coherent set of values, beliefs, norms, and practices of a particular group.
   d. is learned only through formal instruction.

2. In the United States, dominant health attitudes about birth include all of the following *except*
   a. birth is dangerous for mother and infant.
   b. breastfeeding is the optimal way to feed an infant.
   c. breastfeeding is reasonably easy for most mothers.
   d. breastfeeding must be practiced in private.

3. Cultural relativism refers to a(n)

   a. appreciation and acceptance of other cultural norms.

   b. appreciation of one's relatives and how they live and work.

   c. belief that one's own culture is the only right way to live.

   d. recognition that all cultures share the same basic values.

4. A lactation consultant evaluating breastfeeding practices of a client from another culture does *not* need to ask herself whether the practice is

   a. common.

   b. harmful.

   c. harmless.

   d. helpful.

5. An immigrant from Southeast Asia who has children born abroad and born in the United States is *most* likely to

   a. breastfed all of her children.

   b. breastfeed children born abroad but formula-feed those born in the United States.

   c. formula-feed all of her children.

   d. formula-feed children born abroad but breastfeed those born in the United States.

6. Immigrants may formula-feed children born in the United States because of all of the beliefs below *except* a belief that

   a. ancillary dollar costs of breastfeeding are too high.

   b. breastfeeding is outdated or old-fashioned.

   c. formula strengthens children's bones.

   d. traditional parturition rituals, now unavailable to the mother, are needed in order to breastfeed.

7. In 2006 in the United States, lowest rates of breastfeeding were found in _____ women.

   a. African-American, non-Hispanic

   b. Hispanic

   c. Southeast Asian.

   d. white, non-Hispanic.

8. A principal influence guiding an African-American mother after the birth of a child is the

   a. baby's father.

   b. mother's mother.

   c. mother's sisters.

   d. mother's women friends.

9. Interviews with African-American mothers enrolled in WIC programs found that mothers felt that they were offered

   a. insufficient breastfeeding support throughout pregnancy and the early postpartum.

   b. sufficient prenatal education in breastfeeding.

   c. sufficient breastfeeding support postpartum.

   d. sufficient referrals to breastfeeding-support groups in the community.

10. Effective rituals

    a. are beyond the ability of Western science to explain.

    b. have been rigorously analyzed and shown to produce the desired result.

    c. reflect a belief in the efficacy of a particular ceremony.

    d. require adherence to traditional forms.

11. _____ cultures treat colostrum as _____.

    a. Almost all / the accepted first food for a newborn.

    b. Almost no / fit only to be expressed and discarded.

    c. Almost no / "old" or "stale" milk.

    d. Some / a valuable first food whereas others avoid using it.

12. A belief that breastfeeding women may not engage in sexual intercourse (because semen is thought to contaminate breastmilk) is _____, because _____.

    a. harmful to mother and infant / monogamous men may pressure the mother to wean the infant.

    b. helpful to mother and infant / a superimposed pregnancy that would likely impair the health of the current infant is avoided.

    c. helpful to mother and infant / the interval between successive infants increases.

    d. good and bad / all of the above.

13. Sexual relations after childbirth are *best* resumed shortly after which factor is in place?

    a. Father is ready.

    b. Mother is ready.

    c. Parents have agreed on a contraceptive method.

    d. Parents are sleeping through most nights.

14. Secluding a mother and newborn for about 6 weeks (the original "quarantine" of 40 days) generally serves to

    a. allow the mother to focus on her infant and develop a good breastfeeding relationship.

    b. diminish maternal strength by limiting her activity.

    c. impair the infant's immune system because of lack of challenges to his system.

    d. make the baby clingy because he sees so few other people.

15. Which of the following admits of a cultural interpretation?

    a. Age at which the infant is able to digest cereals

    b. Eruption of the first tooth

    c. Some signs of dehydration

    d. Time at which milk comes in

16. To avoid being thought the cause of *mal de ojo* in an Hispanic infant, a lactation consultant should

    a. look at the mother immediately after gazing at the child.

    b. not look the infant in the eyes.

    c. not touch the infant's fontanel.

    d. touch the infant while she admires him.

Discussion Questions

1. What is the definition of *culture?*

2. Are cultural rituals concerning breastfeeding effective? Why or why not?

3. What is the difference between allopathic and folk medicine? What is an example of a belief that typifies each?

4. As you evaluate unfamiliar breastfeeding practices, how might you categorize them in order to focus on which practices to support and which to attempt to modify?

5. What is an example of a common practice that is potentially harmful to a breastfeeding baby? How might you attempt to modify that practice?

6. What might be the underlying physiological reasons for a 40-day period of seclusion after childbirth?

7. What foods have been (or still are) used as galactogogues?

8. How is colostrum viewed in various cultures? Is it always the first food given to a newborn? Why or why not?

9. What reasons might contribute, in the United States, to the generally lower rate of breastfeeding by African-American women?

10. How might the offer of free formula (as in the United States, by the WIC program) affect intention to breastfeed? Would it be ethical to not offer formula at all? What incentives to breastfeed does WIC offer?

11. What beliefs in various cultures influence the use of wet nurses or donor breastmilk?

12. What advantages accrue to an infant who is swaddled and secured to his mother's side or back much of the day?

13. How do cultures that typically consume little meat obtain protein in their diet? What are complementary proteins? How do they figure into the diet?

14. What are some food restrictions or preferences practiced by women in various cultures during the postpartum period? What purposes are served by these restrictions or preferences?

15. What is the basis for categorizing foods as "hot" or "cold"? What cultures categorize foods in this way? How are foods in these categories used to maintain health? How might foods so categorized affect a pregnant or breastfeeding woman?

16. What is the difference between gradual, deliberate, and abrupt weaning? What circumstances might prompt each type of weaning?

17. What developmental milestones are used in various cultures to indicate an appropriate time for weaning a child?

chapter 25

The Familial and Social Context of Breastfeeding

Introduction

It is not just mothers and babies who breastfeed; the entire family breastfeeds in the sense that family members must in various ways accommodate the breastfeeding dyad. For many women, however, the family may be incomplete or a source of danger. Questions in this chapter will help you to assess your understanding of this body of information and how it applies to professional practice.

IBLCE Disciplines

Information in this chapter applies to the following disciplines tested on the certification examination offered by the International Board of Lactation Consultant Examiners: G = Psychology, Sociology, and Anthropology; J = Ethical and Legal Issues.

Multiple-Choice Questions

1. The addition of a baby to a family nearly always _____ family stress, because _____.
    a. decreases / caring for the infant brings the family together.
    b. decreases / parents have a reason for declining requests that impinge on family time.
    c. increases / the baby requires that the family develop new relationships.
    d. increases / the well-being of the baby, rather than themselves, becomes the principal focus.

2. When a second child joins a household consisting of a mother, father, and older sibling, how many pairs of relationships now exist between these four persons?
    a. 10
    b. 6
    c. 4
    d. 3

3. A first-time breastfeeding mother *most* needs which of the following in order to continue breastfeeding?

   a. A healthcare provider who can explain optimal breastfeeding practices

   b. A helper to keep the house in order

   c. Friends who are continuing breastfeeding

   d. Supplementary income to help meet new expenses

4. Significant others who support a mother's breastfeeding efforts usually are

   a. best kept at a distance to avoid them trying to take over care of the baby.

   b. going to try to undermine the closeness of the breastfeeding relationship.

   c. necessary for long-term breastfeeding.

   d. nice but not necessary to continued breastfeeding.

5. The *strongest* predictor of who will initiate and continue breastfeeding is

   a. easily everted nipples.

   b. infant weight at birth—the higher the weight, the longer the duration of breastfeeding.

   c. higher socioeconomic status.

   d. strength of maternal intention to breastfeed.

6. Intention to breastfeed is linked with all of the following *except* maternal

   a. confidence in her ability to breastfeed.

   b. positive attitude toward breastfeeding.

   c. social networks that support her intention to breastfeed.

   d. strong focus on the nutritional benefits of breastfeeding.

7. Research shows that the teaching and advice of a lactation consultant are *most* likely to increase a woman's intention to breastfeed if the mother

   a. hears this information at a prenatal class.

   b. hears this information through a friend.

   c. is undecided about feeding, rather than determined to formula feed.

   d. Only a and b.

   e. Only a and c.

8. The person who usually exerts the most influence on how a woman feeds her infant is

   a. her best friend.

   b. her mother.

   c. the baby's father.

   d. the paternal grandmother.

9. In the early weeks after a child is born, fathers may feel all of the following *except*

   a. ambivalent about the closeness of the mother-infant relationship.

   b. sexual frustration.

   c. pushed aside by the mother.

   d. that it is manly to talk easily about a, b, and c.

10. Fathers can develop a good relationship with their infant, *especially* by
    a. carrying or rocking a baby to console him.
    b. feeding the baby one feeding per day.
    c. insisting on an orderly house as a means to a calm household.
    d. modeling a strong, authoritarian role for his infant.

11. Adolescent mothers in the United States typically breastfeed at lower rates than adult women because they
    a. never even consider breastfeeding.
    b. produce milk with lower nutrient density.
    c. produce smaller volumes of milk so their baby does not gain well.
    d. think that breastfeeding will be both painful and embarrassing.

12. Characteristics linked with mothers who formula-feed their infants include all of the following *except*
    a. age in mid-twenties at birth of first child.
    b. low income.
    c. not married to baby's father.
    d. not finish high school.

13. To effectively assist teenage mothers to breastfeed, a lactation consultant should do all of the following *except*
    a. anticipate the teen mother's needs.
    b. assure the teen that she will not mind figure changes associated with having a new baby.
    c. encourage the teen to ask for needed help.
    d. help the teen mother obtain a breast pump in anticipation of her return to school or job.

14. A low-income woman is more apt to breastfeed if she is characterized by all of the following *except*
    a. she begins prenatal care in the first trimester.
    b. is married to the baby's father, who supports breastfeeding.
    c. left school before 12th grade.
    d. was herself breastfed.

15. Prenatal education classes that thoroughly discuss breastfeeding with low-income black mothers tended to increase all of the following *except*
    a. duration of breastfeeding.
    b. initiation of breastfeeding.
    c. incidence of painful postpartum engorgement.
    d. intention to breastfeed.

16. The step of the Baby-Friendly Hospital Initiative that *least directly* increases duration of breastfeeding is
    a. ample rooming-in—more than 60 percent of the time.
    b. help mothers initiate breastfeeding within 30 minutes after birth.
    c. no use of formula or pacifiers.
    d. referral to community organizations that support breastfeeding.

17. A lactation consultant's *best* role in a legal proceeding to decide custody of a breastfeeding infant is to
    a. advocate for more breastfeeding-friendly laws in her state.
    b. educate herself about the law related to custody of a breastfeeding infant.
    c. educate parents' attorneys about the physical and psychological importance of breastfeeding to the infant's health.
    d. publicize the plight of the breastfeeding mother.

18. A lactation consultant who believes that a client is being physically abused has an obligation to
    a. counsel the mother about how to increase her safety and that of her infant.
    b. overlook evidence of abuse and try to make breastfeeding a bright part of the mother's life.
    c. report her observations to child-protection authorities.
    d. sympathize but limit her actions to breastfeeding advice.

19. As compared with families in which infants are fed formula, families in which infants are breastfed are likely to experience _____ domestic violence toward _____.
    a. less / either women or children.
    b. less / women but not toward children.
    c. more / children but not toward women.
    d. more / women but not toward children.

20. Women who have experienced childhood sexual assaults are _____ likely to _____.
    a. less / initiate breastfeeding.
    b. more / become pregnant as teenagers.
    c. more / delay sexual activity until late adulthood.
    d. more / to bond closely with their infant.

Discussion Questions

1. What can a father do, other than feeding, to grow close to his infant?

2. How does each of the following factors influence the likelihood that a low-income or high-income mother will breastfeed?
   • Access to information about lactation and breastfeeding
   • Degree of support from family, friends, healthcare providers
   • Hospital practices during labor and delivery in the postpartum
   • Racial or ethnic group
   • Use of manufactured baby milks by hospital staff

3. What factors are more likely to deter teenage mothers, as compared with older mothers, from breastfeeding?

4. What differences in breastfeeding behavior have been documented between adolescent and adult mothers?

5. Among low-income women, how does the advice and support provided by peer counselors influence breastfeeding initiation? Duration of exclusive breastfeeding? Total duration of breastfeeding? What makes peer counseling successful in helping women to continue breastfeeding?

6. How may childhood sexual abuse express itself in a woman who states an intention to breastfeed? Are such women more likely or less likely to initiate breastfeeding?

7. Is there a relationship between breastfeeding and maternal feelings of empowerment? If so, what is the relationship? What causes it?

8. In the United States, what obstacles hinder many hospitals from becoming fully "Baby-Friendly"?

Answer Key to Multiple Choice Questions

Chapter 1

1. c
2. b
3. c
4. a
5. d
6. b
7. b
8. a
9. d
10. c
11. a
12. b
13. d

Chapter 2

1. d
2. a
3. b
4. c
5. a
6. b
7. a
8. a
9. a
10. d
11. c

12. c
13. c
14. c
15. a
16. b
17. a
18. d
19. b
20. c
21. c
22. c
23. d
24. a
25. b
26. c
27. c
28. a
29. c
30. c
31. d
32. b

Chapter 3

1. a
2. a
3. c
4. b

5. a
6. a
7. d
8. b
9. d
10. a
11. b
12. f
13. b
14. a
15. c
16. d
17. a
18. d
19. c
20. d
21. d
22. a
23. b
24. b
25. c
26. a
27. d
28. b
29. a
30. a
31. c

32. b
33. d
34. c
35. a
36. b
37. a
38. b
39. c
40. c
41. a
42. d
43. c
44. b
45. b
46. b
47. c
48. a
49. c
50. d
51. c
52. d
53. a
54. d
55. b
56. d
57. c
58. d

59. b
60. a
61. b
62. c
63. d
64. c
65. e
66. d
67. c
68. d
69. b
70. d
71. c

Chapter 4

1. b
2. d
3. b
4. a
5. c
6. d
7. a
8. c
9. d
10. b
11. d
12. c

13. a
14. b
15. c
16. d
17. a
18. c
19. c
20. a
21. b
22. d
23. a
24. c
25. b
26. b
27. c
28. a
29. d
30. a
31. b
32. c
33. b
34. c
35. a
36. e
37. a
38. a
39. a
40. c
41. a
42. b
43. b
44. c
45. c

46. a
47. b
48. d
49. a
50. d
51. c
52. c
53. d
54. d
55. c
56. d
57. a
58. c
59. d
60. b
61. c
62. d
63. b

Chapter 5
1. c
2. d
3. d
4. d
5. a
6. c
7. c
8. b
9. d
10. a
11. b
12. d
13. d

14. b
15. a
16. d
17. b
18. b
19. c
20. a
21. c
22. b
23. a
24. c
25. b
26. b
27. c
28. c
29. a
30. c
31. b
32. a
33. b

Chapter 6
1. a
2. c
3. b
4. c
5. b
6. c
7. b
8. c
9. b
10. b
11. a

12. c
13. a
14. c
15. b
16. c
17. b

Chapter 7
1. c
2. d
3. b
4. d
5. b
6. c
7. d
8. b
9. d
10. a
11. c
12. a
13. d
14. c
15. d
16. a
17. a
18. b
19. a
20. d
21. c
22. d
23. c
24. c
25. d

26. b
27. a
28. d
29. a
30. b
31. c
32. b
33. c
34. a
35. c
36. c
37. c
38. d
39. d
40. a

Chapter 8
1. b
2. c
3. c
4. b
5. c
6. d
7. c
8. a
9. c
10. d
11. c
12. b
13. b
14. a
15. c
16. b

17. e	50. a	16. d	9. b	**Chapter 11**
18. a	51. a	17. b	10. d	1. b
19. d	52. b	18. c	11. d	2. a
20. a	53. a	19. a	12. c	3. d
21. c	54. b	20. e	13. c	4. a
22. a	55. d	21. c	14. d	5. d
23. b	56. a	22. b	15. b	6. a
24. d	57. a	23. c	16. a	7. b
25. a	58. d	24. a	17. d	8. b
26. c	59. a	25. b	18. b	9. b
27. b	60. c	26. a	19. b	10. c
28. b	61. c	27. b	20. c	11. b
29. c	62. b	28. d	21. a	12. d
30. b	63. b	29. d	22. c	13. d
31. a	64. f	30. a	23. c	14. c
32. b	65. d	31. c	24. d	15. d
33. b		32. c	25. d	16. c
34. d	**Chapter 9**	33. a	26. a	17. a
35. b	1. b	34. a	27. a	18. a
36. d	2. a	35. c	28. c	19. b
37. a	3. c	36. d	29. d	20. a
38. b	4. d	37. d	30. a	21. c
39. c	5. a	38. b	31. b	22. a
40. d	6. d		32. b	23. a
41. a	7. d	**Chapter 10**	33. b	24. b
42. d	8. b	1. c	34. d	25. b
43. a	9. b	2. a	35. b	26. d
44. a	10. d	3. d	36. d	27. b
45. b	11. c	4. a	37. b	28. d
46. c	12. c	5. d	38. c	29. b
47. c	13. d	6. b	39. c	30. c
48. c	14. b	7. a	40. b	31. d
49. d	15. b	8. b		32. a

33. c	26. c	14. c	3. b	19. d
34. d	27. b	15. a	4. c	20. c
35. b	28. d	16. a	5. b	21. b
36. c	29. c	17. b	6. c	22. c
37. a	30. c	18. c	7. a	23. b
38. a	31. c	19. b	8. b	24. b
	32. c	20. d	9. d	25. a
Chapter 12	33. b	21. c	10. a	26. c
1. c	34. b	22. a	11. d	27. d
2. d	35. c	23. a	12. b	28. d
3. c	36. c	24. c	13. a	29. a
4. c	37. a	25. b	14. a	30. d
5. d	38. a	26. d	15. d	
6. c	39. d	27. d		**Chapter 16**
7. b	40. b	28. a	**Chapter 15**	1. b
8. c	41. b	29. d	1. d	2. a
9. b	42. a	30. b	2. a	3. d
10. d	43. c	31. d	3. b	4. c
11. a		32. b	4. d	5. b
12. a	**Chapter 13**	33. d	5. d	6. d
13. c	1. b	34. a	6. c	7. a
14. c	2. a	35. b	7. a	8. b
15. c	3. a	36. c	8. c	9. c
16. b	4. d	37. c	9. d	10. d
17. d	5. b	38. d	10. c	11. c
18. b	6. d	39. a	11. d	12. b
19. a	7. c	40. b	12. a	13. b
20. d	8. b	41. b	13. c	14. a
21. d	9. a	42. c	14. a	15. b
22. c	10. d		15. a	16. a
23. d	11. d	**Chapter 14**	16. d	17. b
24. c	12. b	1. a	17. c	18. a
25. d	13. b	2. d	18. a	19. c

20. d

21. a

22. d

23. d

24. b

25. c

26. d

27. c

28. a

29. d

30. a

31. a

32. c

33. d

34. c

35. b

36. b

37. a

Chapter 17

1. b

2. c

3. a

4. a

5. d

6. a

7. b

8. b

9. c

10. b

11. a

12. a

13. c

14. b

15. a

16. b

17. a

18. b

19. a

20. b

Chapter 18

1. b

2. a

3. b

4. b

5. b

6. a

7. c

8. c

9. c

10. b

11. d

12. d

13. b

14. d

15. a

16. c

17. a

18. d

19. b

20. a

21. b

22. c

23. b

24. c

25. c

26. d

27. d

28. a

29. d

30. a

31. d

32. d

33. c

34. b

35. a

36. b

37. d

Chapter 19

1. a

2. c

3. a

4. a

5. d

6. b

7. b

8. c

9. a

10. b

11. d

12. b

13. d

14. b

15. b

16. a

17. b

18. c

19. c

20. d

21. c

22. a

23. d

24. a

25. c

26. c

27. a

28. a

29. d

30. c

31. d

32. b

33. c

34. a

35. d

36. d

37. a

38. b

39. c

40. d

41. c

42. d

43. a

44. c

45. d

46. a

47. b

48. a

49. b

50. c

51. c

52. a

Chapter 20

1. c

2. d

3. a

4. c

5. c

6. a

7. b

8. a

9. b

10. d

11. d

12. b

13. c

14. d

15. a

16. c

17. a

18. d

19. b

20. d

21. a

22. d

23. a

24. d

25. c

26. a

27. d

28. b

29. b

30. d

31. d

32. b

33. d

34. a

35. b

36. d

37. b

38. c

39. c

40. b

Chapter 21

1. a

2. c

3. a

4. a

5. c

6. d

7. d

8. a

9. d

10. c

11. d

12. a

13. b

14. d

15. c

16. b

17. a

18. b

19. d

20. b

21. c

22. d

23. b

Chapter 22

1. a

2. d

3. c

4. d

5. a

6. b

7. c

8. c

9. b

10. a

11. a

12. c

13. d

14. b

15. a

16. d

17. b

18. d

19. a

20. b

21. c

22. b

23. c

24. b

25. a

26. b

27. a

28. c

29. d

Chapter 23

1. c

2. c

3. d

4. a

5. c

6. b

7. a

8. d

9. c

10. d

11. a

12. b

13. d

14. b

15. c

16. b

17. c

18. b

19. c

20. c

21. b

22. b

23. d

Chapter 24

1. c

2. c

3. a

4. a

5. b

6. a

7. a

8. b

9. a

10. c

11. d

12. d

13. b

14. a

15. c

16. d

Chapter 25

1. c

2. b

3. c

4. c

5. d

6. d

7. e

8. c

9. d

10. a

11. d

12. a

13. b

14. c

15. c

16. b

17. c

18. c

19. a

20. b